Communications
in Computer and Information Science   736

Commenced Publication in 2007
Founding and Former Series Editors:
Alfredo Cuzzocrea, Orhun Kara, Dominik Ślęzak, and Xiaokang Yang

More information about this series at http://www.springer.com/series/7899

Carsten Röcker · John O'Donoghue
Martina Ziefle · Markus Helfert
William Molloy (Eds.)

Information and Communication Technologies for Ageing Well and e-Health

Second International Conference, ICT4AWE 2016
Rome, Italy, April 21–22, 2016
Revised Selected Papers

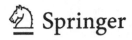 Springer

Editors
Carsten Röcker
Fraunhofer Institute of Optronics, System
  Technology and Image Exploitation
Lemgo
Germany

John O'Donoghue
Imperial College London
London
UK

Martina Ziefle
RWTH Aachen University
Aachen
Germany

Markus Helfert
School of Computing
Dublin City University
Dublin 9
Ireland

William Molloy
Centre for Gerontology
Dublin City University
Cork
Ireland

ISSN 1865-0929   ISSN 1865-0937 (electronic)
Communications in Computer and Information Science
ISBN 978-3-319-62703-8   ISBN 978-3-319-62704-5 (eBook)
DOI 10.1007/978-3-319-62704-5

Library of Congress Control Number: 2017945733

Printed on acid-free paper

This Springer imprint is published by Springer Nature
The registered company is Springer International Publishing AG
The registered company address is: Gewerbestrasse 11, 6330 Cham, Switzerland

Preface

The present book includes extended and revised versions of a set of selected papers from the Second International Conference on Information and Communication Technologies for Ageing Well and e-Health (ICT4AWE 2016), held in Rome, Italy, during April 21–22, 2016.

ICT4AWE 2016 received 39 paper submissions from 22 countries, of which 21% are included in this book. The papers were selected by the event chairs and their selection is based on a number of criteria including the classifications and comments provided by the Program Committee members, the session chairs' assessment, and also the program chairs' global view of all papers included in the technical program. The authors of selected papers were then invited to submit a revised and extended version of their papers having at least 30% innovative material.

The International Conference on Information and Communication Technologies for Ageing Well and e-Health aims to be a meeting point for those that study and apply information and communication technologies for improving the quality of life of the elderly and for helping people stay healthy, independent, and active at work or in their community during the course of their life. ICT4AWE facilitates the exchange of information and dissemination of best practices, innovation, and technical improvements in the fields of age-related health care, education, social coordination, and ambient-assisted living. From e-health to intelligent systems and ICT devices, this is a point of interest for all those who work in research and development and in companies involved in promoting the well-being of aged people, by providing room for industrial presentations, demos, and project descriptions.

The papers selected to be included in this book contribute to the understanding of relevant trends of current research on ageing well and e-health, including: ambient-assisted living, mobile assistive technology, lifestyle engineering and life quality, electronic health records, security and privacy in e-health, smart environments, home care, and remote monitoring.

We would like to thank all the authors for their contributions and also the reviewers who helped ensure the quality of this publication.

April 2017

Carsten Röcker
John O'Donoghue
Martina Ziefle
Leszek Maciaszek
William Molloy

Organization

Conference Co-chairs

Leszek Maciaszek   Wroclaw University of Economics, Poland and Macquarie
University, Sydney, Australia

William Molloy   Centre for Gerontology and Rehabilitation,
School of Medicine, UCC, Ireland

Program Co-chairs

Carsten Röcker   Ostwestfalen-Lippe UAS and Fraunhofer IOSB-INA,
Germany

Martina Ziefle   RWTH-Aachen University, Germany

John O'Donoghue   Imperial College London, UK

Program Committee

Mehdi Adda	Université du Québec à Rimouski, Canada
Carmelo Ardito	Università degli Studi di Bari, Italy
Narcis Avellana	Sensing & Control, Spain
Carlo Alberto Avizzano	Scuola Superiore Sant'Anna, Italy
Christopher Baber	University of Birmingham, UK
Angel Barriga	IMSE-CNM-CSIC, Spain
Karsten Berns	Robotics Research Lab, Germany
Dario Bonino	Istituto Superiore Mario Boella, Italy
Noel Carroll	ARCH, Applied Research for Connected Health Technology Centre, Ireland
Maria Luisa Damiani	Università degli Studi di Milano, Italy
Louise Demers	University of Montreal, Canada
Jinjuan Heidi Feng	Towson University (Baltimore Hebrew University), USA
David Luigi Fuschi	BRIDGING Consulting Ltd., UK
Ennio Gambi	Università Politecnica Delle Marche, Italy
Todor Ganchev	Technical University of Varna, Bulgaria
Jaakko Hakulinen	University of Tampere, Finland
Andreas Heinig	Fraunhofer Institute for Photonic Microsystems, Germany
Alina Huldtgren	Eindhoven University of Technology, The Netherlands
David Kaufman	Simon Fraser University, Canada
Takahiro Kawamura	Toshiba Corp., Japan
Peter Kokol	University of Maribor, Slovenia
Shin'ichi Konomi	University of Tokyo, Japan
Andrej Kos	University of Ljubljana, Slovenia
Mikel Larrea	Universidad del País Vasco, Spain

Linda Little	Northumbria University, UK
Amy Loutfi	Örebro University, Sweden
Hagen Malberg	TU Dresden, Germany
Piero Malcovati	University of Pavia, Italy
Giuseppe Mangioni	Università degli Studi di Catania, Italy
Heimar De Fatima Marin	Universidade Federal de São Paulo, Brazil
Cezary Mazurek	Poznan Supercomputing and Networking Center, Poland
René Meier	Lucerne University of Applied Sciences, Switzerland
Hiroshi Mineno	Shizuoka University, Japan
Iosif Mporas	University of Hertfordshire, UK
Amit Anil Nanavati	IBM Research, India
Anthony F. Norcio	University of Maryland Baltimore County, USA
John O'Donoghue	Imperial College London, UK
Helen Pain	University of Edinburgh, UK
Marcelo Pimenta	UFRGS, Brazil
Marco Porta	Università degli Studi di Pavia, Italy
Ulrich Reimer	University of Applied Sciences St. Gallen, Switzerland
Philippe Roose	LIUPPA/IUT de Bayonne/UPPA, France
Zafer Sahinoglu	Mitsubishi Electric Research Laboratories, USA
Corina Sas	Lancaster University, UK
Sreela Sasi	Gannon University, USA
Fabio A. Schreiber	Politecnico di Milano, Italy
Jitae Shin	Sungkyunkwan University, Korea, Republic of
Josep Silva	Universitat Politècnica de València, Spain
Kostas Stathis	Royal Holloway University of London, UK
Yin-Leng Theng	Nanyang Technological University, Singapore
Gerhard Weber	Technical University of Dresden, Germany
Nadir Weibel	University of California, USA
Robert Woitsch	Boc Asset Management, Austria
George Xylomenos	Athens University of Economics and Business, Greece

Additional Reviewers

Christos Antonopoulos	University of Patras, Greece
Martin Franke	TU Dresden, Germany
Urban Sedlar	University of Ljubljana, Slovenia

Invited Speakers

Hubert Österle	Institute of Information Management (IWI), University of St. Gallen, Switzerland
Margaret Ross	Southampton Solent University, UK

Contents

Supporting Caregivers in Nursing Homes for Alzheimer's Disease Patients: A Technological Approach to Overnight Supervision

Laura Montanini[1(✉)], Laura Raffaeli[1], Adelmo De Santis[1],
Antonio Del Campo[1], Carlos Chiatti[2], Luca Paciello[3], Ennio Gambi[1],
and Susanna Spinsante[1]

[1] Dipartimento di Ingegneria dell'Informazione,
Università Politecnica delle Marche, Ancona, Italy
l.raffaeli@univpm.it
[2] Italian National Research Centre on Ageing (INRCA), Ancona, Italy
[3] ArieLAB S.r.l., Ancona, Italy

Abstract. The reduction of public expenditure and investments in health care provisioning calls for new, sustainable models to transform the increasing aging population and dementia-related diseases incidence from global challenges into new opportunities. In this context, Information and Communication Technologies play a vital role, to both promote aging in place and home management of Patients with Dementia, and to provide new tools and solutions to facilitate the working conditions of the care staff in nursing homes, which remain an essential facility when cognitive-impaired patients cannot live at home anymore. Night staff in nursing homes are a vulnerable group, receiving less supervision and support than day staff, but with high levels of responsibility. Additionally, nighttime attendance of patients affected by dementia may be difficult, because of their incremented neuropsychiatric symptoms. This paper describes an integrated system for the night monitoring of patients with dementia in nursing homes, based on a product originally conceived for domestic use, but re-designed to provide support to nurses, by means of a set of sensors located in each patient's room, and suitable software applications to detect dangerous events and raise automatic alerts delivered to the nurses through mobile devices. The results obtained from the first experimental installation of the monitoring system proved the effectiveness of the proposed solution to support nurses during the night supervision of patients, and suggested suitable modifications and additional features to increase the nurses' compliance.

Keywords: Environmental sensors · Unobtrusive monitoring · Activity detection · Alarm notification · Behavioral analysis

1 Introduction

It is widely recognized that Information and Communication Technologies (ICT) have the potential to dramatically impact social and welfare systems in

© Springer International Publishing AG 2017
C. Röcker et al. (Eds.): ICT4AWE 2016, CCIS 736, pp. 1–19, 2017.
DOI: 10.1007/978-3-319-62704-5_1

promoting new economically viable and sustainable models for healthcare delivery, especially when targeting the aging populations, and, among them, Patients with Dementia (PwDs) and their caregivers. By 2050, 22% of the world's population will be over 60 years of age [26], and both governments and the private sector need to mobilize innovation and research to transform this global challenge into an opportunity for new models of sustainable growth. Among the chronic diseases that mostly affect aging population, Dementia and Alzheimer's Disease (AD) have a prominent role [4]. ICT offers several opportunities to health services, specifically to PwDs and their caregivers, as discussed in a systematic review by Martínez-Alcalá et al. [22]. The paper shows that among the 26 studies that satisfied the inclusion criteria for the review, 16 were aimed at the PwDs, and 10 at the primary caregivers and/or family members. Basically, it means that the current literature almost neglects the opportunities ICT can offer to formal caregivers of PwDs, like professionals and healthcare operators, and to nurses working in the residential care sector. On the other hand, it is known since long time that professional caring of PwDs may have strong impacts on the carer's physical and mental health [12]; at the same time, improvements in nursing home residents' quality of life may be achieved by enhanced training and deployment of the care workers [33].

Staff working in care and nursing homes is typically undersized with respect to the real workload, because of budgetary restrictions on the amount of personnel that can be recruited, compared to the number of patients cared after. This results in a stressful working condition, as many tasks need to be carried out in a relatively short time. Since 2010, due to the global economic crisis, growth in public health spending came almost to a halt across the OECD (Organisation for Economic Cooperation and Development) members, with even reductions in many countries [28]. Anyway, despite the current trend of promoting elderly caring at home and aging in place, the role of nursing homes remains relevant, especially for PwDs or AD patients at an advanced stage, who cannot be assisted at home anymore. ICT should be more extensively exploited to facilitate the working conditions of the care staff dealing with PwDs, and to improve the quality of care, but the impact of technology on the underlying long-term established clinical work processes needs to be carefully evaluated and analysed. Possible blocks in the execution of routine procedures, due to the adoption of technology, tend to distract staff from care issues, and may lead to new errors. Typically, in reaction to this condition, nurses develop problem-solving behaviors that bypass the use of new technology, or adapt the work process so as to minimize disruption in traditionally executed procedures [5,13,20].

The so-called "sundown syndrome" in PwDs is characterized by the emergence or increment of neuropsychiatric symptoms such as agitation, confusion, anxiety, and aggressiveness in late afternoon, in the evening, or at night, probably due to impaired circadian rhythm, environmental and social factors, and compromised cognition [16]. Although night-time care forms a significant part of care provision in nursing homes, little research has focused on this. Night staff are a vulnerable group, receiving less training, supervision and support than day staff, but with high levels of responsibility [10]. Several ICT-based solutions have been proposed to facilitate home-caring of people affected by dementia or AD during the night hours. In fact, nighttime activity is a common occurrence in persons with dementia, which increases the risk for injury and unattended home exits, and impairs the sleep patterns of caregivers [17,18]. Technology has been applied to develop tools that alert caregivers of suspicious nighttime activity, to help prevent injuries and unattended exits [21,27,32]. Nighttime attendance of patients affected by dementia or AD may be difficult to manage also in nursing homes, especially because the number of nurses available is reduced, with respect to daily hours. As a consequence, it is of interest to evaluate the applicability of technology for night monitoring of AD patients in nursing homes, in order to assess the impact of technology on nurses' work flows, and on the quality of assistance provided to patients.

This paper describes an integrated system for the monitoring of AD patients, realized by evolving and updating an already existing product named UpTech [7]. The UpTech project focused on AD patients and their family caregivers; it was carried out as a multi-component randomized clinical trial (RCT), integrating previous evidence on the effectiveness of AD care strategies, in a comprehensive design, to reduce the burden of family caregivers of AD patients, and to maintain AD patients at home. Indeed, often the relatives who take care of AD patients are subjected to high levels of stress, that could also contribute to the onset of physical problems. The positive outcomes of the UpTech experimental phase [30], providing the use of technological devices as alternative or complementary form of support, have suggested its application in a different scenario, represented by the nursing homes. The aim of the new project, named UpTech RSA [24], is to support and help assistance of AD patients in nursing homes, during the night hours, by means of a set of sensors located in patients' rooms, and suitable software applications to detect dangerous events and raise alerts for the nurses.

When dealing with *monitoring* of people, this condition is often seen as violating the privacy of the user. Therefore, in order to satisfy the requirement of providing an unobtrusive monitoring, only simple environmental sensors have been employed in the UpTech RSA solution, that are less intrusive and more acceptable than other options, like wearable devices, or video cameras. Wireless sensors have been chosen and used: on one hand, this enables a simple installation, on the other hand, power consumption is a critical aspect, which has to be evaluated at the design stage.

The paper is organized as follows: the context of application of the proposed technology is discussed in Sect. 2, whereas Sect. 3 is focused on design and deployment issues. The field trial implementation is presented in Sect. 4, and the results gathered from the practical use of the technology in a real nursing home are discussed in Sect. 5, showing how the data collected from sensors may be translated into useful information for understanding the patients' needs and requirements. Finally, Sect. 6 concludes the paper and suggests possible future developments.

2   Context

Dementia is becoming increasingly prevalent worldwide and is today considered as one of the most burdensome disease for the developed societies. AD is the most common form of degenerative dementia. Generally, the onset of the illness occurs in the pre-senile age, however it could be even earlier. A person with dementia can live 20 years or more after diagnosis, during which he/she experiences a gradual change of the functional and clinical profile. As a consequence of the disease, a progressive loss of cognitive capacity is occurring, eventually leading to disability and to a severe deterioration of quality of life. During the so-called "dementia journey", the disease affects not only the patients but also their informal (e.g. families) and formal (e.g. care staff) caregivers, on whom the bulk of the care burden falls [8].

Up-to-date, there is no cure for dementia thus the attention to the symptomatic non-pharmacological treatment for the patients and their caregivers has become increasingly relevant, especially as the literature shows that these can be more effective that most of the available drugs [31]. Although home remains the preferred place for care delivery, a substantial number of patients need to access (permanently or temporarily) residential care facilities, when home care is no longer feasible. In the residential context, infrastructure and staffing levels are not always adequate to manage residents with dementia. Residential care services are indeed labour intensive and the quality of care here depends largely on the staffing level and characteristics [15, 23]. As the ongoing financial crisis is reducing the budget available for residential care services, a detrimental effect on personnel standards might occur. This concrete risk of staff shortcomings might, in turn, lead to a substantial proportion of avoidable hospitalisations, use of emergency departments, increased carers' burden and stress, and inappropriate use of chemical and physical restraints (e.g. antipsychotics).

The literature suggests that education, training and support of available staff, supervision, and improvement of job satisfaction could be effective measures to increase quality of care in assisted care settings [14]. In addition, technologies and other environmental factors have been identified as the most promising measures to improve working conditions in the residential care setting, to reduce the care burden and to improve the overall quality of care [2, 11]. The potentials of new technologies have been tested to reduce the need for continuous monitoring of dementia patients, and to increase their safety and well being within the residential setting.

Aloulou et al. [1] describe the development and deployment of an Ambient Assisted Living (AAL) system for nursing homes. They have tested the system, comprising a set of environmental sensors, devices to enable interaction and a centralized machine for each room, involving 8 patients and their caregivers, in a nursing home in Singapore. Field trials are extremely important: in this case for example, the installation outside a laboratory environment led to recognize problems derived from the real usage. Secondly, the first test phase conducted only with caregivers enabled a preliminary evaluation of the system and its refining without affecting the patients. Finally, the complete test provided an overall description of the system capabilities, its effectiveness, the benefits brought to the patients and the caregivers, the contribution to improve the quality of the assistance provided and to support the caregivers.

Several solutions can be found in the literature that adopt assistive technologies (ATs) to help PwDs at home, to perform the usual daily tasks and thus to maintain their independence. As for the type of ATs adopted, a mapping study have been conducted, based on literature and industrial (limited to UK market) surveys [3]. From this research, 5 main types of ATs have been identified: robotics, health monitoring, prompts and reminders, communication, software. Moreover, it seems that there is a gap between academic research and industrial products, since the literature mainly focuses on robotics and health monitoring, while the UK industry mainly develops health monitoring and software based technologies.

Other papers affirm that reminding technologies are an active area of research. Patterson et al. [29] provide an overview of works addressed to this topic, but they also find out that often the adherence to these reminders is not considered. They start from the principle that the user acknowledge is not sufficient to assess the real execution of the task following the reminder: therefore, they propose a prototype that integrates reminders and adherence detection, along with the possibility to inform a carer in case of non-compliance.

Despite the rich literature on the available technologies, there are a few studies that involve PwDs in determining the results of using ATs [9]. Most of them include people with mild and moderate dementia but often the stage of the disease is not specified. As for the assessment of the quality of life, a standard approach is necessary to carry out a significant comparison across studies.

3 Design and Deployment

The system described in this paper represents an evolution of a project named UpTech, aimed at improving the quality of life of both AD patients living at home and their family caregivers. This project involved nurses and social workers, who periodically went to the patients' houses, and included the installation of technological kits at the patients' homes. Each kit consisted of a network of wireless sensors installed in the house, for the monitoring of the patient. Data were processed by a central control unit and, in case of danger, a notification was sent to the caregiver. The new system, called UpTech RSA, targets the nursing home environment and has been devised primarily for the overnight monitoring of patients, when there is a lack of personnel in the building. Moreover, the main differences between the two systems concern the following aspects:

- number of users: in the nursing home, multiple patients are monitored at the same time. Thus, the central control unit is able to manage data coming from more than one set of sensors;
- sensors: different types of sensors are employed, due to the diversity of the physical environment;

– system architecture: the whole network can be seen as a set of sub-networks, one for each room;
– alarm management: the monitoring system is an aid for the nurses, the notifications are not sent to the remote caregiver as in the home-based system.

The project development stage carried out in the Laboratory was aimed first at the improvement of the previous UpTech kit, secondly at the design and implementation of the modules required for the new system. In particular, the radio transceivers firmware was re-designed, to implement an efficient data acquisition and transmission procedure. At the same time, particular attention was paid to the energy consumption exhibited by the transmission nodes, by taking into account the values of power absorption in the different operation phases, and implementing all the possible strategies for its reduction. As for the new components, the following modules have been designed: the structure of the database used to store the collected information, and the applications necessary to implement the decision algorithms, in charge of making actions depending on particular values of the acquired data.

The system requirements have been identified by collecting nurses' requests, thus the developed functionalities are related to the usual daily care procedures. Specifically, the set of sensors installed in each room enables the following functionalities:

– door opening detection;
– window opening detection;
– "French-window" opening detection;
– presence in bed detection;
– presence in the bathroom detection.

The door opening detection is achieved using a magnetic sensor, wireless connected by Sub-GHz technology at a frequency of 868 MHz to a gateway, by means of a properly designed electronic equipment.

Similarly, the detection of windows opening is obtained through the same technology (see Fig. 1[1]). The user's presence in the bathroom is detected by a self-powered Passive Infrared Sensor (PIR), which is connected to the radio transmitter module. For ease of installation, and to avoid damage to the fixtures of the building, these sensors have been placed on top of the entry doors of the bathrooms. A mat sensor has been adopted to detect the user's presence in bed; it is available in two versions, with and without self-calibration. The sensor without self-calibration is placed over the mattress, under the sheets, while the other one is placed under the mattress (Fig. 2), and therefore it results more comfortable for the patients and for the daily operations of bed maintenance. The gateway represents a central node that forwards data to a PC located at the nurses' station. Then, the application running on the PC filters the incoming information. Data related to events are saved in a local database (DB), while those referred to the operating status of the sensors are verified in order to monitor the correct operation of the technology kits.

---

[1] All figures in the paper are reproduced from [24].

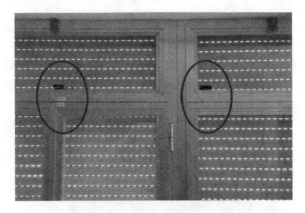

Fig. 1. Magnetic sensors for windows opening detection.

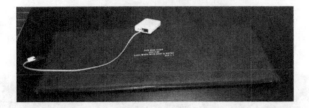

Fig. 2. Self-calibrating mat sensor, for under-the-mattress positioning.

The electronic boards transmit an event to the central server every time there is a status change, that is, for example, activation/deactivation of the PIR sensor, or opening/closing the door. Accordingly, the data stored in the database contain the sensor information (id, gateway address, name and type), the date and time when the notified event occurred, and the status of the sensor represented in binary format as follows:

- activation: *state* = 1;
- deactivation: *state* = 0.

In addition, the server assigns a unique id to each DB row in order to implement a robust mechanism for transmitting information to the mobile interface. This allows the mobile device to identify one or more missing events, and to request them back from the server. In fact, a mobile Android application has been developed, running on a tablet or smartphone, and so easily portable. This allows the nursing staff to receive event notifications even when they are outside the nurses' station and cannot access the fixed desktop interface. Events data, properly processed, are displayed through not only mobile, but also desktop interfaces (Figs. 3 and 4). In the first case, the user can see a scrollable list of events identified by the name of the sensor that generated it and the room name, as shown in Fig. 3. Each event is tagged with a colored circle: depending

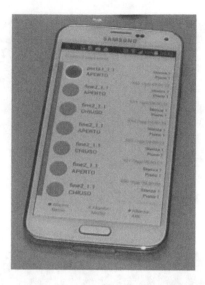

Fig. 3. Mobile interface running on a smartphone.

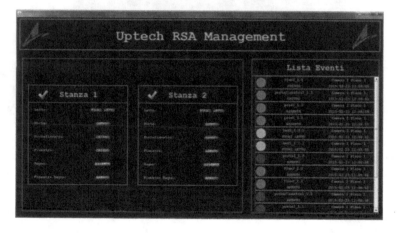

Fig. 4. Screenshot of the Desktop Interface, *two sections* version. (Color figure online)

on the associated level of alert, the circle may be green, yellow or red. In the latter case, two versions are available:

- a *two sections* version: the graphic interface is organised into two parts. On the right there is a scrollable list of the events acquired by the sensors, while on the left the status of the sensors in each room is shown. There is a top bar which becomes coloured and flashing when an event occurs;
- a *multi-user* version: the main screen shows all the rooms monitored. When an event occurs in one room, the corresponding frame becomes colored. By clicking on the box, it is possible to see the details of sensors state.

Given the wireless transmission mode of the sensor nodes and their battery supply, the monitoring of the sensors state itself becomes very important. Therefore, a procedure for the periodic sending of alive messages has been implemented in the sensors. They are constantly monitored by the central processing system, that generates alarm messages in the case of failure. Despite its importance, this procedure is extremely critical, because sending *alive* messages too frequently causes an increase in the batteries consumption. Otherwise, the transmission of the *alive* message at a lower frequency can give rise to long time intervals in which the sensor is not active, but the system is not informed about the failure. When an *alive* message does not reach the local server at the expected time, the latter notifies a malfunction of the sensor node to the nurse, who can promptly find out the problem and act accordingly.

4   Field Trial

4.1   Experimental Set-up

The system described in Sect. 3 is already available as a prototype. Following the initial development phase in the Laboratory, aimed to better adapt the technology to the emerged operational requirements, the prototype has been installed in the nursing home "Villa Cozza" in Macerata (Italy). In this phase, the supervision of two rooms (tagged as room 2 and room 3) has been implemented, while the final version of the system will be able to dynamically accept a plurality of rooms, depending on the operating requirements. Each room is equipped with a sensors kit consisting of three magnetic sensors (one applied onto the window, one onto the French window, and one onto the room front door), a PIR sensor in the bathroom, and a force sensor placed in the bed, as shown in Fig. 5. A single gateway device has been used to manage wireless communications with the sensors in the two rooms.

In room 2 two female patients are housed, only one suffering from AD. Her bed has been equipped with a force sensor. The other one is not autonomous and can move only by a wheelchair; consequently, the events generated by the different sensors can be originated only by the movement of the first patient. In room 3, instead, a single female patient is housed, also suffering from AD, but in this case she can not move autonomously. As the system represents a support tool for improving the safety of patients, it can be well-compared to an alarm system. Moreover, the type of sensors employed do not collect personal data of the two patients involved. According to the national laws, in this case the ethical approval is not required.

During the installation phase, it has been critical to enable the communication between the gateway, positioned in the corridor in front of the two rooms, and the central server, located in the nurses' station on the upper floor. Such a problem arises because the building where the nursing home is located is not equipped with a communication infrastructure (e.g. a Local Area Network): there are no network cables, or WiFi coverage. Moreover, the nursing home is hosted in a historic building and, as often happens in such cases, the walls are thick

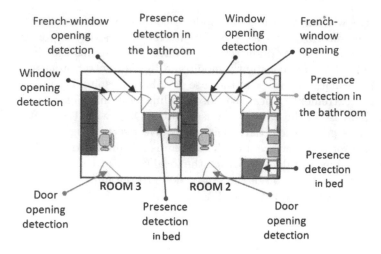

Fig. 5. Floor plan of the two rooms equipped with the UpTech RSA sensors in the nursing home "Villa Cozza", Macerata (Italy).

and made of concrete, thus making wireless communications very difficult. Both a Power Line Communication (PLC) and a mixed wireless infrastructure (WiFi and Hiperlan) have been experimented, finally selecting the wireless solution as the supporting communication architecture. In order to overcome obstacles like metal doors and thick walls, that limit signal propagation, multiple Access Points (APs) and links have been setup.

4.2   Evaluation Survey

Some weeks after the installation a survey for the evaluation of the system has been conducted over 18 nurses. Although some of them are not very familiar with the technology, the results are highly positive. In Table 1, some of the most significant questions and results are listed. The 100% of respondents believes the kit is easy to use and recommends it for the monitoring of AD patients in nursing homes during the night. All the nurses state the system has not been a source of stress for them. In fact, its introduction does not generate further work for the staff. They just carried on the usual activities, but with an additional monitoring tool. Only 6% of the nurses believes that it was stressful for patients. Indeed, operators have received some sporadic grumbles due to the discomfort produced by one of the bed sensors. As mentioned in Sect. 2, the bed force sensor without calibration must be placed between mattress and sheet: this may annoy the patient during sleep time, due to a difference in thickness. This leads us to conclude that the sensor with calibration is preferable, as it can be placed under the mattress, and will be consequently used in the subsequent installations. Apart from that, patients did not notice any change.

Moreover, the nurses stated that, during the trial period, there have been some dangerous episodes detected by the kit, such as the opening of a window

Table 1. The opinion of the nurses about the experimental deployment of the UpTech RSA technology at the nursing home "Villa Cozza".

Question	Yes	No	
Is the kit easy to use?	100%	0%	
Do you think that the patients monitored have suffered a stress?	6%	94%	
Do you think that the kit has been a source of stress for nurses?	0%	100%	
Would you recommend the use of this kit in nursing homes?	100%	0%	
Question	Positive	Medium	Negative
Overall opinion on the technological kit	89%	11%	0%
Question	Yes	Quite a lot	No
Do you think that the kit can improve the assistance provided in nursing homes?	61%	39%	0%

during the night, and a patient's fall out of the room. In both cases the system detected the alarming situation and the staff was able to intervene promptly. Despite the positive opinions, some problems were found, in particular due to the occurrence of false alarms. They were caused primarily by failures in the communication link, resulting in multiple sending of alarm events.

Still considering nurses' opinions, some ideas for improving the system were identified. First, false alarms must be avoided, as they can generate a feeling of distrust by operators against the entire system. Secondly, customizing different alarms for each user would be preferable, since each patient has different behavioural and health conditions. Finally, implementing an even more friendly user interface would encourage the adoption of the system by nurses unfamiliar with technology.

5   Data Analysis

5.1   Context Characterization

In addition to the real-time monitoring of patients, it is possible to perform several types of analysis on the data collected by UpTech RSA sensors over time, such as obtaining information on the patient's habits and, as a consequence, detecting any changes or unusual behaviours. In the following, some sample graphs are shown, representing selected daily activities of the monitored patients, obtained thanks to the events detected by the sensors. The analysis refers to data collected from May to June, 2015, by the sensors located in both the monitored rooms.

First of all, in order to give significance to the analysed data, some information about the patients and the daily activities conducted in the Alzheimer's ward are necessary. Table 2 represents a sort of daily diary. Patients remain within the ward during the day: they can stay together in the common areas, where they also have lunch and dinner, and can go in/out of the rooms whenever they want. The entry doors of the rooms are generally closed during the night. They are opened by the shift nurse who performs two inspection rounds per night, in order to verify that the patients are sleeping and do not need assistance.

Table 2. Diary of daily activities.

Time	Activity
7:30	Rooms cleaning
7:00–10:00	Patients get out of beds
Morning	Patients stay in the common areas, can go in/out of the rooms
11:30–12:30	Lunch in the dining room
Afternoon	Patients stay in the common areas, some of them have a rest
17:30–18:30	Dinner in the dining room
19:00–21:00	Patients go to bed
22:00	First nurses' check round
3:00	Second nurses' check round

In room 2 there are two patients: only one is monitored through a bed sensor, because she suffers from AD and often wakes up in the night and goes out of the room. The other patient moves by wheelchair and is not able to get off the bed on her own. The AD patient in room 3 has bed rails, so she can not get out of the bed autonomously during the night.

Although the system is able to monitor the patients throughout the entire day, the interesting events are those occurring during the night. In that period, in fact, the user is left alone for most of the time and thus the data acquired are more significant. The graphical visualization of the analysis output provided in the following sub-section has the ability to help the reader in recognizing and understanding a large amount of data, and in easily identifying anomalies and behavioural patterns that would not be obvious otherwise.

5.2   Data Representation and Analysis

The raw data collected by the sensors installed in the rooms are often difficult to interpret. Therefore, in order to carry out the data analysis, first of all it is necessary to find a representation allowing to understand them immediately. Lotfi et al. [19] affirm that, among the various representation methods presented in the literature, the start-time/duration is the most effective one for large data sets. The data acquired from each sensor can be seen as a binary signal, in which the value "1" is the activation and the value "0" is the deactivation. Representing information according to a start-time/duration method means converting the binary signal into two separate sequences of real numbers corresponding to the start-time and duration of each activity, respectively. Figure 6 shows the start-time/duration graphs of the activity detected by the bed sensor, i.e. presumably sleeping, for each room. Each point on the graph indicates a "sleep" and is characterized by a start-time (on the abscissa) and a duration (on the ordinate). All activities lasting less than 10 min have been ignored because they could indicate sensor activations and deactivations due to involuntary movements of the subject while asleep.

Looking at the charts it is easy to notice the triangular shape assumed by the set of points. This result was expected because life in the nursing home is scheduled by the daily diary and, thus, the sleeping activities are bounded by specific and almost fixed time constraints. Therefore, it seems plausible that patients never go to bed before 6:30 PM, and the sleep duration is inversely proportional to the start-time. The sparse distribution of points in the triangular-shape diagrams indicates that the monitored subject wakes up several times during the night. In Fig. 6(b) a group of points is located between 12:30 PM and 1:30 PM: this suggests that sometimes the patient has a rest after lunch. On the other hand, looking at Fig. 6(a), the presence of two outliers (highlighted by red circles) becomes immediately evident.

Analytically, a first detection of outliers is performed using clustering techniques. In the present case the K-means algorithm is applied [25], which allows condensing the data. Different techniques can be used to separate normal data and outliers [6]. In this case, a variation of the threshold filtering method has been chosen: it consists in both comparing a specific feature of the points with a threshold and excluding the outliers. Specifically, for each cluster identified, and for each point in the cluster, the considered feature is the euclidean distance between one point and the others belonging to the same cluster. Such distances are then compared against a threshold empirically chosen. all points whose distance exceeds the threshold are considered outliers. Moreover, to improve the clustering effect, another iteration of the algorithm is performed, by excluding the abnormalities found from the dataset. Clustering is employed as a pre-processing method, and it can be considered as the basic level of data analysis. It does not provide a definitive result, in fact its application to the dataset has the only aim to help understanding data by means of a graphical representation.

Another information that can be extrapolated by combining the data obtained from the bed sensor with those detected by other sensors, is the identification of the action carried out after the user came out of bed. This will enable the possibility to calculate the occurrences of predefined patterns of activities, instead of single ones. Such an analysis allows to identify potentially dangerous situations with respect to behaviours commonly exhibited by the subject, and not considered as alarms. Each point on the graphs in Fig. 7 indicates a "sleep" and is characterized by a start-time (on the abscissa) and an end-time (on the ordinate). As for the start-time/duration, the start-time/end-time representation requires the conversion of the binary signal in two separate sequences of real

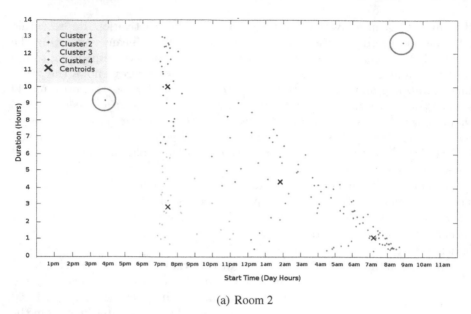

(a) Room 2

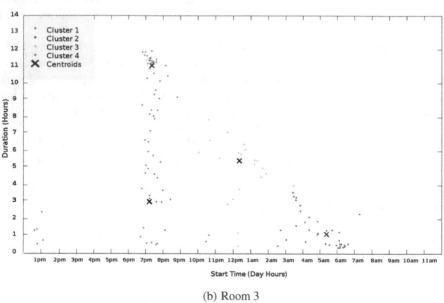

(b) Room 3

Fig. 6. Start-time/duration graphs of the "sleeping" activity detected from May to June 2015, respectively in (a) room 2, and (b) room 3. (Color figure online)

numbers which in this case correspond to the start-time and end-time of the activity. The type of activity shown is still the sleeping, but, according to the action carried out subsequently, the shape and colour of the marker changes.

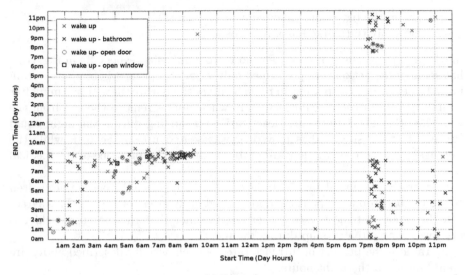

(a) Room 2

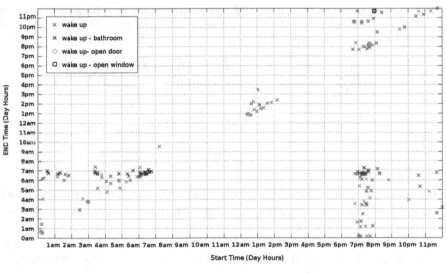

(b) Room 3

Fig. 7. Start-time/end-time graphs representing the activities performed after waking up by the patients housed respectively in (a) room 2, and (b) room 3, from May to June 2015. (Color figure online)

In fact, the graphs show, for each room, the actions executed within 4 min after the patient got out from bed (end-time), i.e.:

- door opening (marked as a green circle);
- window opening (marked as a black square);

– presence in the bathroom (marked as a blue cross);
– no other activity (marked as a red cross).

This kind of representation has been chosen to emphasize, especially in Fig. 7(b), that some of the actions are performed only when the patient gets up at certain times. For example, the patient in room 3 enters the bathroom within 4 min after waking up only in the morning, i.e. only when nurses remove the rail from the bed. The other activations and deactivations occurring during the night could indicate that the subject has moved or was seated up on the bed, while the openings of the door or window are probably due to the presence of the medical staff.

Conversely, looking at Fig. 7(a), the observer can notice the patient very often goes to the bathroom or opens the door immediately after getting up. This agrees with the reports of the nurses concerning the fact that the monitored elder is very lively, and often gets up during the night.

In Table 3, the percent occurrence rates of each activity described above are given, limited to the night hours.

Table 3. Hit rate of the getting up action followed respectively by the action of entering the bathroom, opening/closing the door, or opening/closing the window, in the time slot between 09:00 PM and 06:00 AM.

Event detected after awakening	Room 2	Room3
Presence in the bathroom	76%	15%
Door opening	14%	2%
Window opening	0%	0.2%
None	10%	82.8%

The analysis described so far is just the very first step to identify the user's behavioural patterns and abnormal situations. Until now, we focused on the representation and visualization of data, extracting some preliminary information on the habits of two monitored patients. Nevertheless, there is still a long way to go. Although the detection of outliers can be very useful in this context, however, it is necessary to set up a predictive system able to identify in advance any anomalous situation to help the nursing home staff making the necessary arrangements. As already hinted, one of the aspects emerged during discussion with nurses is the need of alarm personalization. In fact, a situation may be potentially dangerous for a user, while it may be harmless for another one. This strongly depends on motor and cognitive skills of each patient. Although this can be done manually by nurses via graphical user interfaces, a significant contribution comes from the analysis of patients' habits. One of the future developments is to extend the behavioural analysis in the long term, aimed at recognizing unusual, and, therefore, potentially dangerous situations and notifying them to the staff, in a completely automatic way.

6   Conclusion

The comparison of the results obtained from the first experimental installation of the proposed monitoring system to the work already cited in [1], concerning the adoption of an assistive technological system in a nursing home, motivates a number of comments about the outcomes of the research herein presented. First, even if the solution presented in [1] is more complete than ours, we found some basic similarities that confirm the validity of our proposal, such as the choice of adopting wireless environmental sensors, and the usefulness of an overnight assistance. Second, the same referenced paper confirmed that data gathered from non-intrusive sensors can be exploited to perform a long-term analysis on the trend of the patient's conditions. Finally, we learned that before involving patients in the adoption of a new technology targeted to their assistance, this should be tested only with caregivers and nurses. This way, possible malfunctions or false alarms will not affect the patients and will be detected and solved beforehand. Nurses' compliance in using the proposed technology could grow even more by extending the pool of monitored patients, as being able to cover all of them increases the perceived benefit for the nurses and, above all, the degree of safety of the patients.

Acknowledgements. This work was partially funded through an Innovation Voucher issued in the framework of the WIDER project (Green Growing of SMEs: Innovation and Development in the Energy Sector in the Med Area), and partially by the AAL 2014-1-041 project "Home4Dem" (HOME-based ICT solutions FOR the independent living of people with DEMentia and their caregivers), co-founded by the Active and Assisted Living Joint Platform.

References

1. Aloulou, H., Mokhtari, M., Tiberghien, T., Biswas, J., Phua, C., Lin, J.H.K, Yap, P.: Deployment of assistive living technology in a nursing home environment: methods and lessons learned. BMC Med. Inform. Decis. Mak. **13**(1), 42 (2013). doi:10.1186/1472-6947-13-42
2. Ancker, J.S., Witteman, H.O., Hafeez, B., Provencher, T., de Graaf, M.V., Wei, E.: The invisible work of personal health information management among people with multiple chronic conditions: qualitative interview study among patients and providers. J. Med. Internet Res. **17**(6), e137 (2015). doi:10.2196/jmir.4381
3. Asghar, I., Cang, S., Yu, H.: A systematic mapping study on assitive technologies for people with dementia. In: 2015 9th International Conference on Software, Knowledge, Information Management and Applications (SKIMA), pp. 1–8, December 2015
4. Alzheimer's Association: 2016 alzheimer's disease facts and figures. Alzheimer's Dementia **12**(4), 459–509 (2016). http://www.alz.org/documents_custom/2016-facts-and-figures.pdf
5. Bowens, F.M., Frye, P.A., Jones, W.A.: Health information technology: integration of clinical workflow into meaningful use of electronic health records. Perspect. Health Inf. Manage./AHIMA, Am. Health Inf. Manage. Assoc. **7**, 1d (2010). http://europepmc.org/articles/PMC2966355

6. Chandola, V., Banerjee, A., Kumar, V.: Anomaly detection: a survey. ACM Comput. Surv. **41**(3), 15: 1–15: 58 (2009). http://doi.acm.org/10.1145/1541880. 1541882

7. Chiatti, C., Masera, F., Rimland, J., Cherubini, A., Scarpino, O., Spazzafumo, L., Lattanzio, F.: The up-tech project, an intervention to support caregivers of alzheimer's disease patients in Italy: study protocol for a randomized controlled trial. Trials **14**(1), 155 (2013). doi:10.1186/1745-6215-14-155

8. Chiatti, C., Rimland, J.M., Bonfranceschi, F., Masera, F., Bustacchini, S., Cassetta, L.: The up-tech project, an intervention to support caregivers of alzheimer's disease patients in Italy: preliminary findings on recruitment and caregiving burden in the baseline population. Aging Mental Health **19**(6), 517–525 (2015)

9. Cook, G.A., Bailey, C., Moyle, W.: The impact of ICT-based telecare technology on quality of life of people with dementia: review of the literature. In: 2013 6th International Conference on Human System Interactions (HSI), pp. 614–619, June 2013

10. Kerr, D., Wilkinson, H., Cunningham, C.: Supporting older people in care homes at night (2008). https://www.jrf.org.uk/report/supporting-older-people-care-homes-night

11. Freedman, V.A.: Barriers to implementing technology in residential long-term care settings. Polisher Research Institute (2005)

12. Hallberg, I.R., Norberg, A.: Nurses' experiences of strain and their reactions in the care of severely demented patients. Int. J. Geriatr. Psychiatry **10**(9), 757–766 (1995). doi:10.1002/gps.930100906

13. Huston, C.: The impact of emerging technology on nursing care warp speed ahead. OJIN Online J. Issues Nurs. **18**(2), 1 (2013)

14. Institute of Medicine: Improving the Quality of Care in Nursing Homes. The National Academies Press, Washington, DC (1986). http://www.nap.edu/catalog/646/improving-the-quality-of-care-in-nursing-homes

15. Kahanpää, A., Noro, A., Finne-Soveri, H., Lehto, J., Perälä, M.L.: Perceived and observed quality of long-term care for residents - does functional ability account? Int. J. Older People Nurs. (2016). doi:10.1111/opn.12110

16. Khachiyants, N., Trinkle, D., Son, S.J., Kim, K.Y.: Sundown syndrome in persons with dementia: an update. Psychiatry Invest. **8**(4), 275–287 (2011). http://doi.org/10.4306/pi.2011.8.4.275

17. Kim, S.S., Oh, K.M., Richards, K.: Sleep disturbance, nocturnal agitation behaviors, and medical comorbidity in older adults with dementia: relationship to reported caregiver burden. Res. Gerontol. Nurs. **7**(5), 206–214 (2014). doi:10.3928/19404921-20140512-01

18. Lee, D., Heo, S.H., Yoon, S.S., Chang, D.I., Lee, S., Rhee, H.Y., Ku, B.D., Park, K.C.: Sleep disturbances and predictive factors in caregivers of patients with mild cognitive impairment and dementia. J. Clin. Neurol. **10**(4), 304 (2014). doi:10.3988/jcn.2014.10.4.304

19. Lotfi, A., Langensiepen, C., Mahmoud, S., Akhlaghinia, M.: Smart homes for the elderly dementia sufferers: identification and prediction of abnormal behaviour. J. Ambient Intell. Hum. Comput. **3**(3), 205–218 (2012). doi:10.1007/s12652-010-0043-x

20. Lowry, S.Z., Ramaiah, M., Patterson, E.S., Brick, D., Gibbons, M.C., Paul, L.A.: Integrating electronic health records into clinical workflow: an application of human factors modeling methods to specialty care in 'obstetrics and gynecology' and 'ophthalmology'. Technical report, National Institute of Standards and Technology (2015). doi:10.6028/NIST.IR.8042

21. Mao, H.F., Chang, L.H., Yao, G., Chen, W.Y., Huang, W.N.W.: Indicators of perceived useful dementia care assistive technology: caregivers' perspectives. Geriatr. Gerontol. Int. **15**(8), 1049–1057 (2015). doi:10.1111/ggi.12398
22. Martínez-Alcalá, I.C., Pliego-Pastrana, P., Rosales-Lagarde, A., Lopez-Noguerola, J., Molina-Trinidad, M.E.: Information and communication technologies in the care of the elderly: systematic review of applications aimed at patients with dementia and caregivers. JMIR Rehabil. Assist. Technol. **3**(1), e6 (2016). http://rehab.jmir.org/2016/1/e6/
23. Milte, R., Shulver, W., Killington, M., Bradley, C., Ratcliffe, J., Crotty, M.: Quality in residential care from the perspective of people living with dementia: the importance of personhood. Arch. Gerontol. Geriatr. **63**, 9–17 (2016). doi:10.1016/j.archger.2015.11.007
24. Montanini, L., Raffaeli, L., Santis, A.D., Campo, A.D., Chiatti, C., Rascioni, G., Gambi, E., Spinsante, S.: Overnight supervision of alzheimer's disease patients in nursing homes: system development and field trial. In: 2016 2nd International Conference on ICT for Ageing Well, April 2016
25. Nazerfard, E., Rashidi, P., Cook, D.: Discovering temporal features and relations of activity patterns. In: 2010 IEEE International Conference on Data Mining Workshops (ICDMW), pp. 1069–1075, December 2010
26. Obi, T., Auffret, J., Iwasaki, N.: Aging Society and ICT: Global Silver Innovation, 1st edn. IOS Press, Amsterdam (2013)
27. Occhiuzzi, C., Vallese, C., Amendola, S., Manzari, S., Marrocco, G.: Night-care: a passive RFID system for remote monitoring and control of overnight living environment. Procedia Comput. Sci. **32**, 190–197 (2014). The 5th International Conference on Ambient Systems, Networks and Technologies (ANT-2014), The 4th International Conference on Sustainable Energy Information Technology (SEIT-2014). http://www.sciencedirect.com/science/article/pii/S1877050914006140
28. Organization for Economic Co-operation and Development. Focus on health spending: OECD health statistics 2015 (2015). http://www.oecd.org/health/health-systems/Focus-Health-Spending-2015.pdf
29. Patterson, T., et al.: Home-based self-management of dementia: closing the loop. In: Geissbühler, A., Demongeot, J., Mokhtari, M., Abdulrazak, B., Aloulou, H. (eds.) ICOST 2015. LNCS, vol. 9102, pp. 232–243. Springer, Cham (2015). doi:10.1007/978-3-319-19312-0_19
30. Pombo, N., Spinsante, S., Chiatti, C., Olivetti, P., Gambi, E., Garcia, N.: Assistive technologies for homecare: outcomes from trial experiences. In: ICT Innovations 2015 Proceedings, Workshop ELEMENT 2015 (2015)
31. Spijker, A., Vernooij-Dassen, M., Vasse, E., Adang, E., Wollersheim, H., Grol, R., Verhey, F.: Effectiveness of non pharmacological interventions in delaying the institutionalization of patients with dementia: a meta-analysis. J. Am. Geriatr. Soc. **56**(6), 1116–1128 (2008). doi:10.1111/j.1532-5415.2008.01705.x
32. Vuong, N.K., Goh, S.G.A., Chan, S., Lau, C.T.: A mobile-health application to detect wandering patterns of elderly people in home environment. In: 2013 35th Annual International Conference of the IEEE Engineering in Medicine and Biology Society (EMBC), pp. 6748–6751. Institute of Electrical & Electronics Engineers (IEEE) (2013). doi:10.1109/EMBC.2013.6611105
33. Zimmerman, S., Sloane, P.D., Williams, C.S., Reed, P.S., Preisser, J.S., Eckert, J.K., Boustani, M., Dobbs, D.: Dementia care and quality of life in assisted living and nursing homes. Gerontol. **45**(suppl 1), 133–146 (2005). http://gerontologist.oxfordjournals.org/content/45/suppl_1/133.abstract

Monitoring Activities of Daily Living Using Audio Analysis and a RaspberryPI: A Use Case on Bathroom Activity Monitoring

Georgios Siantikos$^{(\boxtimes)}$, Theodoros Giannakopoulos, and Stasinos Konstantopoulos

Institute of Informatics and Telecommunications, NCSR Demokritos, Athens, Greece
{dickos,tyianak,konstant}@iit.demokritos.gr

Abstract. A framework that utilizes audio information for recognition of activities of daily living (ADLs) in the context of a health monitoring environment is presented in this chapter. We propose integrating a Raspberry PI single-board PC that is used both as an audio acquisition and analysis unit. So Raspberry PI captures audio samples from the attached microphone device and executes a set of real-time feature extraction and classification procedures, in order to provide continuous and online audio event recognition to the end user. Furthermore, a practical workflow is presented, that helps the technicians that setup the device to perform a fast, user-friendly and robust tuning and calibration procedure. As a result, the technician is capable of "training" the device without any need for prior knowledge of machine learning techniques. The proposed system has been evaluated against a particular scenario that is rather important in the context of any healthcare monitoring system for the elder: In particular, we have focused on the "bathroom scenario" according to which, a Raspberry PI device equipped with a single microphone is used to monitor bathroom activity on a 24/7 basis in a privacy-aware manner, since no audio data is stored or transmitted. The presented experimental results prove that the proposed framework can be successfully used for audio event recognition tasks.

Keywords: Audio analysis · Activities of daily living · Health monitoring · Remote monitoring · Audio sensors · RaspberryPI · Audio event recognition

1 Introduction

Although fully autonomous artificial intelligence is actively researched and advanced, the current state of the art (and at the level of maturity required for commodity electronics) has machine learning methods rely on delicate training and configuration sessions in order to adapt to different environments. When embedding machine learning methods in commodity electronics this is typically worked around by uploading the signal and receiving analysis results from remote

© Springer International Publishing AG 2017
C. Röcker et al. (Eds.): ICT4AWE 2016, CCIS 736, pp. 20–32, 2017.
DOI: 10.1007/978-3-319-62704-5_2

centralized services. Recent examples include voice-operated personal assistant applications and companion, toy, and "pet" applications.

This model, however, suffers from its obvious privacy implications. These implications are further exacerbated in the telemedicine domain for two reasons: the data collected by the remote service is not only more sensitive, but the users might also not be able to make informed decisions or might not be offered reasonable alternatives. Home monitoring for the elderly is a prime example: the increase in life expectancy and in the need for long-term care creates a pressure to seek alternatives to institutional healthcare for the aged population. Advancements in robotics and automation and in artificial intelligence and intelligent monitoring are explored as a way to prolong independent living at home while providing guarantees of safety and adequate medical monitoring [1–3]. The users of such solutions, however, might be suffering from mild cognitive impairment or be unable to afford conventional monitoring, which makes ethically questionable any consent they provide to upload and analyse raw content of their activities of daily living (ADL) in order to extract medical monitoring information. Several methods have been used to detect activities of daily living in real home environments, focusing on elderly population ([4–7]) and a wide range of modalities.

In this paper, we present an audio analysis system (Sect. 2) that explores the integration of the audio sensor and the processing unit as Raspberry PI[1] device. Such a unit is able to execute signal processing and machine learning algorithms in order to eliminate the need to provide raw content: the only information that leaves the confines of the integrated unit is an abstract ADL log. Although such information still needs to be managed in full accordance to guidelines pertaining private data, the level of obtrusiveness is greatly reduced by the assurance that no unwarranted analysis or recording can conceivably be done.

Our system is designed to satisfy two key requirements: that the analysis algorithms are computationally efficient so that they can be implemented for the Raspberry PI device; and that they can be tuned and configured for different acoustic environments by technicians without machine learning expertise. In order to evaluate the proposed approach on these requirements, we motivate and present a use case based on bathroom usage (Sect. 3) and draw conclusions (Sect. 3).

2 Proposed Method

2.1 Overall Architecture

The main part of the whole system is a microphone-equipped Raspberry PI single-board PC that is used for all data acquisition and processing. Its small-form factor, low energy consumption and low overall cost make it ideal for installing it in any room/area we want to monitor and its processing power is enough for running our algorithms in real time. In our experiments we used a Raspberry PI model B with a Wolfson audio card.

---

[1] Please cf. https://www.raspberrypi.org.

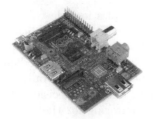

Fig. 1. The Raspberry PI device.

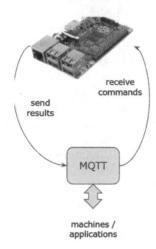

Fig. 2. MQTT-based messaging communication.

Communication to/from the PC is made using the MQTT machine-to-machine communication protocol. MQTT is a lightweight messaging protocol that implements the brokered publish/subscribe pattern, created widely used in IoT applications. Without going into technical details, the main idea is that when connected to a specified MQTT broker, various machines/applications can send messages under a certain topic and others can listen to these when "subscribed" to these topics. In our use case, it is used both for sending commands to the Raspberry PI (for example to start/stop recording) and for remotely receiving the processing results (Fig. 1).

For this purpose, two MQTT clients were implemented: The first is installed in the Raspberry PI and is subscribed to a "command" topic in order to receive requests for collecting training data, building audio classes models and finally use them for real-time classification. The second one is bundled in an Android application and is used for sending remotely the corresponding commands and listening to the classification results. The system is designed with ease of use in mind and the only set-up needed is connecting the two clients to the same broker. By having a dedicated broker this step can be performed automatically, making the whole system plug-and-play (Fig. 2).

2.2   System Calibration

Once setup, the system has to go through a training phase in order to be used for real-life scenarios. This includes recording, feature extraction, manual annotation of the recorded events and classifier tuning/training. Figure 3 shows the proposed calibration procedure. During this phase, the various events are recorded using the Android application as a remote controller of the Raspberry PI device that makes the actual recording and further processing. An audio file is created on user's demand and the user/technician is informed about the categories and durations of already recorded data. He then provides the current recording's label (e.g. "door bell").

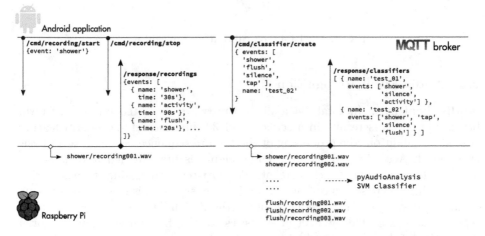

Fig. 3. From left to right: User initiates an event recording and the corresponding file is created. When user stops, a response is returned with information about the events recorded so far. When a reasonable amount of data is gathered, an SVM classifier for the desired events can be created using the pyAudioAnalysis library. In this case, the response contains information about the classifiers available for future use. Reproduced from [8].

When a reasonably large amount of data is gathered (typically about 1–2 minutes of recordings for each category), the technician uses the mobile application to trigger the training process (that is also executed on the Raspberry PI device). After this process, the Raspberry PI is ready to monitor and recognize sound in the "learned" environment. This conceptual sequence of steps for the calibration procedure is also visualized in Fig. 4.

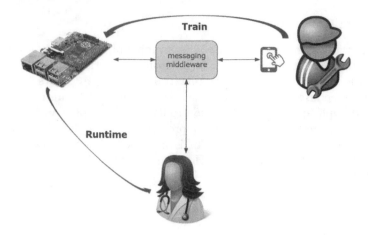

Fig. 4. MQTT-based calibration procedure.

2.3   Audio Event Recognition

Audio Features. In total, 34 audio features are extracted on a short-term basis. This process results in a sequence of 34-dimensional short-term feature vectors. In addition, the processing of the feature sequence on a mid-term basis is adopted. According to that the audio signal is first divided into mid-term windows (segments). For each segment, the short-term processing stage is carried out and the feature sequence from each mid-term segment, is used for computing feature statistics (e.g. the average value of the ZCR). Therefore, each mid-term segment is represented by a set of statistics. In this Section we provide a brief description of the adopted audio features. For detailed description the reader can refer to the related bibliography [9–11]. The time-domain features (features 1–3) are directly extracted from the raw signal samples, while the frequency-domain features (features 4–34, apart from the MFCCs) are based on the magnitude of the Discrete Fourier Transform (DFT). The cepstral domain (e.g. used by the MFCCs) results after applying the Inverse DFT on the logarithmic spectrum. The complete list of features is presented in Table 1.

Classification. As described in Sect. 2.3, the feature extraction process leads to a 68-dimensional feature vector for each 1-second audio segment, i.e. 2 statistics × 34 short-term features. Each unknown audio segment of fixed size (1 s in our case) is therefore represented by a 68-D feature vector. Each of these samples is classified using a Support Vector Machine with probabilistic output. We have selected to use probabilistic SVMs [12] due to their ability to generalize well especially in high dimensional classification problems [13]. The model is trained using a cross-validation procedure to select the optimal SVM parameter, namely the soft margin parameter C.

Table 1. Adopted short-term audio features.

Index	Name	Description
1	Zero Crossing Rate	Rate of sign-changes of the frame
2	Energy	Sum of squares of the signal values, normalized by frame length
3	Entropy of Energy	Entropy of sub-frames' normalized energies. A measure of abrupt changes
4	Spectral Centroid	Spectrum's center of gravity
5	Spectral Spread	Spectrum's second central moment of the spectrum
6	Spectral Entropy	Entropy of the normalized spectral energies for a set of sub-frames
7	Spectral Flux	Squared difference between the normalized magnitudes of the spectra of the two successive frames
8	Spectral Rolloff	The frequency below which 90% of the magnitude distribution of the spectrum is concentrated.
9–21	MFCCs	Mel Frequency Cepstral Coefficients: a cepstral representation with mel-scaled frequency bands
22–33	Chroma Vector	A 12-element representation of the spectral energy in 12 equal-tempered pitch classes of western-type music
34	Chroma Deviation	Standard deviation of the 12 chroma coefficients

Audio Analysis Implementation. Audio feature extraction and classification has been implemented using the pyAudioAnalysis library [14]. This is an open-source Python library that implements a wide range of audio analysis functionalities and can be used in several applications. Using pyAudioAnalysis one can classify an unknown audio segment to a set of predefined classes, segment an audio recording and classify homogeneous segments, remove silence areas from a speech recording, estimate the emotion of a speech segment, extract audio thumbnails from a music track, etc. In this work, pyAudioAnalysis has been used to extract audio features, to train the classification models and to perform cross validation experimentation in order to extract the respective performance measures. pyAudioAnalysis achieves $2 \times$ realtime performance on the Raspberry devices, which validates its usage in the context of the particular setup.

3 Bathroom Use Case and Evaluation

3.1 Use Case and Motivation

As discussed in the introduction, the motivating use case for our approach is medical monitoring. Specifically, we base our evaluation setup on allowing elderly people with mild cognitive impairment to maintain an independent life, at their own home, for longer than what is safely possible today.

In order to have a guideline about what information is used by medical doctors to assess such conditions, we use the interRAI Long-Term Care Facilities Assessment System (interRAI LTCF). interRAI LTCF enables comprehensive, standardized evaluation of the needs, strengths, and preferences of persons receiving care. interRAI has been analysed previously in order to identify assessment items, such as mood and ADL logs, that can be automatically recognized and are useful to medical personnel [15]. Among the assessment items listed, we identified those regarding bathroom use as being closest to our concept: these items can be extracted by processing very sensitive content, and being able to provide guarantees about the management and processing of this content would have significant impact on the acceptance of any relevant solution by users.

In this context, we have recorded and manually annotated sounds from bathroom usage. In particular, the following audio classes are trained and evaluated by the proposed methodology:

- Silence - no sound
- Flushing water
- Shower
- Tap water
- Other activities

Note that the selected audio events are location-specific and therefore the adopted calibration workflow can be used during the installation phase, as described in Sect. 2.2.

3.2 Dataset

In order to train and evaluate the proposed event recognition methodology, we have recorded and manually annotated (using the mobile app described earlier in the paper) an audio dataset. The total duration of the dataset is almost 1 hour. The audio recordings and the respective ground truth is openly available at https://iit.demokritos.gr/~tyianak/bathroomScenarioEventsNew.zip

Two different bathroom locations have been used for recording/annotation. This gives us the opportunity to evaluate the performance of the proposed classification method when the respective models have been trained in a different setup. In particular, the complete dataset consists of the following parts:

- A large training dataset of more than 400 audio *segments* to be used for the scenario of the "static" training, according to which, the classifiers are trained beforehand. Note that this subset only consists of audio segments as it is only used for training.
- A subset of 4 audio (continuous) recordings and respective ground-truth annotations. The total duration of this set is 7 min. This dataset is used both for training and testing

3.3   Experimental Evaluation

Performance Measures. Let CM be the confusion matrix, i.e. a $N_c \times N_c$ matrix (N_c is the total number of audio classes), whose rows and columns refer to the true (ground truth) and predicted class labels of the dataset, respectively. In other words, each element, $CM(i, j)$, stands for the number of samples of class i that were assigned to class j by the adopted classification method. The diagonal of the confusion matrix captures the correct classification decisions ($i = j$). CM is normalized row-wise, in order to discard the information that is related to the size of each class:

$$CM_n(i, j) = \frac{CM(i, j)}{\sum_{n=1}^{N_c} CM(i, n)} \tag{1}$$

Obviously, after the normalization process, the elements of each row sum to unity.

Three useful performance measures are then extracted from the confusion matrix. The first is the overall accuracy, Acc, of the classifier, which is defined as the fraction of samples of the dataset that have been correctly classified:

$$Acc = \frac{\sum_{m=1}^{N_c} CM(m, m)}{\sum_{m=1}^{N_c} \sum_{n=1}^{N_c} CM(m, n)} \tag{2}$$

Apart from the overall accuracy, we have adopted two class-specific measures that describe how well the classification algorithm performs on each class. The first of these measures is the class recall, $Re(i)$, which is defined as the proportion of data with true class label i that were correctly assigned to class i:

$$Re(i) = \frac{CM(i, i)}{\sum_{m=1}^{N_c} CM(i, m)} \tag{3}$$

where $\sum_{m=1}^{N_c} CM(i, m)$ is the total number of samples that are known to belong to class i. In addition, we use the class precision ($Pr(i)$), i.e. the fraction of samples that were correctly classified to class i if we take into account the total number of samples that were classified to that class:

$$Pr(i) = \frac{CM(i, i)}{\sum_{m=1}^{N_c} CM(m, i)} \tag{4}$$

Finally, the F_1-measure is also computed, which is the harmonic mean of the precision and recall values:

$$F_1(i) = \frac{2Re(i)Pr(i)}{Pr(i) + Re(i)} \tag{5}$$

Results. Two categories of experiments have been conducted:

- 1st experimental setup: This is the proposed setup, according to which one or more sequences (i.e. the recordings of the second subset of the dataset described in Sect. 3.2) are used to train the classifiers, through the presented mobile interface. The rest of the recordings is used for evaluation.
- 2nd experimental setup: This setup is used for comparison. The idea here is to adopt a "static" model trained from irrelevant data, i.e. segments that have not been recorded and annotated through the mobile interface.

Table 2 shows the (row-wise normalized) confusion matrix and the respective precision, recall and $F1$ measures for each audio class and for the *1st experimental setup*. This is the result of the evaluation process when only one recording is used during the training phase.

Table 2. *1st experimental setup*: Single-recording training: Row-wise normalized confusion matrix, recall precision and F1 measures. Overall F1 measure: 68.1%.

Confusion matrix (%)					
True ⇓	Predicted				
	Shower	Flush	Tap	Silence	Activity
Shower	89.4	1.8	3.0	0.1	5.8
Flush	7.2	70.7	0.4	2.1	19.6
Tap	5.7	4.0	85.8	0.8	3.6
Silence	1.4	4.0	0.0	58.0	36.5
Activity	13.0	11.6	2.6	31.2	41.6
Performance measurements (%, per class)					
Recall:	89.4	70.7	85.8	58.0	41.6
Precision:	76.6	76.8	93.5	62.9	38.8
F1:	82.5	73.6	89.5	60.3	40.2

These results correspond to the most realistic and less demanding (in terms of calibration-training time). In addition, Table 3 demonstrates the ability of the classifiers to adopt to more data, if they can be available. In particular, Table 3 shows the same performance measures if a "leave one out" process is used in the evaluation process, using the described dataset. That is, if three whole recordings are used for each training phase. Results indicate an almost 5% performance boosting. However, using three recordings instead of one means a 300% increase in the calibration time to be carried out by the technicians.

Finally, in Table 4 we present the comparison of the performances of the two experimental setups. The second experimental setup (i.e. the one based on large pre-trained audio datasets) has been evaluated for three different classification approaches, namely: Hidden Markov Models, Convolutional Neural Nets and

Table 3. *1st experimental setup*: Three-recording training: Row-wise normalized confusion matrix, recall precision and F1 measures. Overall F1 measure: 73.8%.

Confusion matrix (%)					
True ⇓	Predicted				
	Shower	Flush	Tap	Silence	Activity
Shower	85.6	1.6	2.6	0.2	10.0
Flush	5.7	86.5	0.0	1.5	6.3
Tap	5.2	3.7	85.5	0.7	4.9
Silence	0.1	3.4	0.0	72.5	24.0
Activity	5.8	9.7	1.5	29.0	53.9
Performance measurements (%, per class)					
Recall	85.6	86.5	85.5	72.5	53.9
Precision	83.6	82.5	95.4	69.8	54.4
F1:	84.6	84.5	90.2	71.1	54.2

Support Vector Machines. On the other hand, only SVMs are used for the proposed approach (i.e. the 1st experimental setup), since it would not make sense to use the other two approaches which, by nature, require more training data. The results prove that, indeed, using location-specific audio data for training the models leads to better classification performance, compared to pretrained models, even if much larger datasets have been used.

Table 4. Performance results for both experimental setups. It is obvious that, regardless of the classification method, using a "static" model that has been trained using external data leads to poor classification performance.

Experimental setup	Method	Performance F_1
1st	1 train	68
	N-1 train	74
2nd	HMM	57
	CNN	59
	SVM	58

4   Conclusions

This paper has presented an architectural approach that employs a Raspberry PI device both as an audio acquisition and analysis unit, in the context of a health monitoring system. The overall goal of such system is to detect and recognize Activities of Daily Living (ADLs) in real living environments of elderly people. Both real-time audio feature extraction and classification methods have been implemented and integrated on the device. Apart from the audio analytics procedures implemented on Raspberry PI, we propose a workflow for a fast and easy-to-use calibration procedure. According to this, the implemented classifiers are actually trainned in the particular home's sound conditions, through a series of simple calibration steps, executed through an Android application, handled by the technician that installs the device. In that way, no requirements for knowledge on machine learning are needed.

Experimental evaluation has demonstrated a 70% classification performance even if a single recording (1 to 1.5 min long) is used in the training process. In addition, experimental evaluation has shown that there is an actual need for a fast and easy retraining procedure. The complete software that was used for the experiments can be found in the project's Git repository[2] under an open-source license.

The proposed system architecture satisfies three vital requirements.

- First, by using computationally efficient algorithms, we manage to cover the needs of data acquisition and processing using only a low-spec'ed Raspberry PI device, while achieving a $2 \times$ realtime performance. This validates the system's suitability in the context of a *low-cost* health monitoring setup as it does not require a workstation or a PC (e.g. [16]), but a single Raspberry PI that serves both as an acquisition and an analysis module. In particular, the total cost of both the acquisition and analysis modules is less than 100$.
- In addition, the system achieves a satisfactory classification performance, given (a) the low-end hardware used and (b) the lack of demand for big training data. Although our method does not outperform (in terms of overall classification accuracy) other similar methods for ADL recognition in the context of a smart home environment, the significant differences in terms of overall cost and easiness of setup, can make the proposed approach preferable for real house applications. For instance, the approach in [17] achieves a 85% classification accuracy in a ADL recognition task, however the acquisition scenario requires multiple microphone sensors and therefore much higher cost.
- The setup procedure (i.e. configuration and calibration of the overall system) for different acoustic environments and target events can be performed by technicians without machine learning expertise. The need for a fast and easy procedure for training the audio classifiers, without any prior knowledge for machine learning methods has been met and the effectiveness of the procedure has been validated through experimental results.

Our ongoing and future research work focuses on the following directions:

- Extend the calibration procedure so that it also takes into account a "base dataset", i.e. an initial classification scheme that is tuned in the context of the annotation process and not re-trained from scratch.
- Use long-term temporal knowledge to smooth the results of the classifier, based on prior knowledge regarding the events.

---

[2] https://bitbucket.org/radioprojectanalysis/ict4awe2016.

Acknowledgements. This project has received funding from the European Union's Horizon 2020 research and innovation programme under grant agreement No 643892. Please see http://www.radio-project.eu for more details.

References

1. Barger, T.S., Brown, D.E., Alwan, M.: Health-status monitoring through analysis of behavioral patterns. IEEE Trans. Syst. Man Cybern. Part A Syst. Hum. **35**, 22–27 (2005)
2. Hagler, S., Austin, D., Hayes, T.L., Kaye, J., Pavel, M.: Unobtrusive and ubiquitous in-home monitoring: a methodology for continuous assessment of gait velocity in elders. IEEE Trans. Biomed. Eng. **57**, 813–820 (2010)
3. Mann, W.C., Marchant, T., Tomita, M., Fraas, L., Stanton, K.: Elder acceptance of health monitoring devices in the home. Care Manage. J. **3**, 91 (2002)
4. Vacher, M., Portet, F., Fleury, A., Noury, N.: Development of audio sensing technology for ambient assisted living: applications and challenges. In: Digital Advances in Medicine, E-Health, and Communication Technologies, p. 148 (2013)
5. Vacher, M., Portet, F., Fleury, A., Noury, N.: Challenges in the processing of audio channels for ambient assisted living. In: 12th IEEE International Conference on e-Health Networking Applications and Services (Healthcom), pp. 330–337. IEEE (2010)
6. Costa, R., Carneiro, D., Novais, P., Lima, L., Machado, J., Marques, A., Neves, J.: Ambient assisted living. Ubiquitous Computing and Ambient Intelligence, pp. 86–94. Springer, Heidelberg (2009)
7. Botia, J.A., Villa, A., Palma, J.: Ambient assisted living system for in-home monitoring of healthy independent elders. Expert Syst. Appl. **39**, 8136–8148 (2012)
8. Siantikos, G., Giannakopoulos, T., Konstantopoulos, S.: A low-cost approach for detecting activities of daily living using audio information: a use case on bathroom activity monitoring. In: Proceedings of the International Conference on Information and Communication Technologies for Ageing Well and e-Health, pp. 26–32 (2016)
9. Giannakopoulos, T., Pikrakis, A.: Introduction to Audio Analysis: A MATLAB® Approach. Academic Press (2014)
10. Theodoridis, S., Koutroumbas, K.: Pattern Recognition, 4th edn. Academic Press, Inc. (2008)
11. Hyoung-Gook, K., Nicolas, M., Sikora, T.: MPEG-7 Audio and Beyond: Audio Content Indexing and Retrieval. Wiley, Chichester (2005)
12. Platt, J.C.: Probabilistic outputs for support vector machines and comparisons to regularized likelihood methods. In: Advances in large margin classifiers, Citeseer (1999)
13. Chapelle, O., Haffner, P., Vapnik, V.N.: Support vector machines for histogram-based image classification. IEEE Trans. Neural Networks **10**, 1055–1064 (1999)
14. Giannakopoulos, T.: pyAudioAnalysis: Python audio analysis library: feature extraction, classification, segmentation and applications (2015). Accessed 27 Apr 2015

15. RADIO Project: D2.2: Early detection methods and relevant system requirements (2015). http://radio-project.eu/deliverables
16. Chen, J., Kam, A.H., Zhang, J., Liu, N., Shue, L.: Bathroom activity monitoring based on sound. In: Gellersen, H.-W., Want, R., Schmidt, A. (eds.) Pervasive 2005. LNCS, vol. 3468, pp. 47–61. Springer, Heidelberg (2005). doi:10.1007/11428572_4
17. Vuegen, L., Van Den Broeck, B., Karsmakers, P., Vanrumste, B., et al.: Automatic monitoring of activities of daily living based on real-life acoustic sensor data: a preliminary study. In: Fourth workshop on speech and language processing for assistive technologies (SLPAT): Proceedings, Association for Computational Linguistics (ACL), pp. 113–118 (2013)

Assessing Ehealth Readiness Within the Libyan National Health Service by Carrying Out Research Case Studies of Hospitals and Clinics in Both Urban and Rural Areas of Libya

Mansour Ahwidy[1,2(✉)] and Lyn Pemberton[1]

[1] School of Computing, Engineering and Mathematics, University of Brighton, Mithras House,
Lewes Road, Brighton, UK
{Ma195,Lp22}@brighton.ac.uk
[2] University of Sabha, Sabha, Libya

Abstract. This research study is conducted to assess Ehealth readiness within the Libyan national health services by carrying out research case studies of hospitals and clinics in both urban and rural areas of Libya. The outcome results will help constructing framework for Ehealth implementation in the Libyan National Health Service (LNHS). The research study assessed how prescription were prescribed, information communication technology (ICT) was used in recording healthcare information, patients were referred, how healthcare staff carry out their consultations, and how they were trained to use IT. This research study was carried out in Zawia, Misrata, Sirt, Benghazi, Tripoli and Sabha healthcare institutions and was focused upon both five urban and rural area and explored the readiness levels of the technical, political, healthcare and social factors that need to be examined when healthcare information systems are planned. Qualitative interviews and quantitative questionnaires were formulated for this research and used the Chan framework (2010) for their formulations. Data were managed using NVIVO for interviews and an SPSS statistical package for Questionnaires. The findings from this research indicated that there was no evidence of Ehealth technology in the LNHS found by the researcher and insufficient IT support and staff ICT training. These results from the rural and urban healthcare institutions place them on the Ehealth Maturity Curve at the interaction and presence stages (level zero). Thus it is essential for specific Ehealth frameworks to be created that are based around these findings for moving the Ehealth technology usage in these healthcare institutions from 0 to 2 in the E-Health Maturity Curve levels.

Keywords: Technology readiness assessment · Ehealth · Patient electronic health records · Electronic prescription

1 Introduction

When Ehealth systems are incorporated in healthcare systems they can support them in addressing the healthcare problems that are now facing most countries within the developing world (Kwankam 2004; Ludwick and Doucette 2009; Lau et al. 2011). However,

© Springer International Publishing AG 2017
C. Röcker et al. (Eds.): ICT4AWE 2016, CCIS 736, pp. 33–48, 2017.
DOI: 10.1007/978-3-319-62704-5_3

in order to introduce Ehealth systems in developing countries there needs to be an overhaul of the ICT systems being used there at present and these calls for examinations of the infrastructure, organisation and political situations in these countries (Hossein 2012). The research carried out on transforming the LNHS has indicated that a majority of Libyans do not have enough access to the basics required for healthcare and most people receive medical attention purely from the LNHS. The LNHS has invested large amounts of money in both urban and rural healthcare institutions and services, along with ICT, in order that the provision of healthcare services are improved by healthcare staff having more efficient work processes (Hamroush 2014). However, although there had been a large financial has been invested, many healthcare staff have not benefitted from improved ICT. This study looks at how Ehealth systems can lead to healthcare professionals carrying out their jobs more effectively and efficiently in the LNHS. For achieving this, the researcher conducted a study of urban and rural healthcare institutions in order to assess their Ehealth readiness and to be able to create an Ehealth framework for improving the job processes of healthcare staff. The study looked at ways in which Ehealth systems could be utilised for improving the keeping of patient healthcare records, making consultations, carrying out training, making referrals and prescribing medication (Bilbey and Lalani 2013; Yellowlees 2005; Broens et al. 2007; Khoja et al. 2007a). This study has lead to the compilation of an Ehealth framework formulated from the research data and it has formulated a list of recommendations that can be utilised for the transition from the present ICT levels in the LNHS to a more complex and developed one where Ehealth solutions can be integrated.

2   The Theory of Ehealth Readiness Assessments

The theory of Ehealth Readiness Assessments was carried out to define Ehealth systems, how they might benefit a populace in a developing country and how the readiness of that country might be evaluated. There are many factors determining the readiness of a country for the implementation of Ehealth systems (Khoja et al. 2007b; Jennett et al. 2004), so it was a rewarding task to investigate the findings of previous research. Using the Brighton University data base, Science Direct, Google Scholar, various Libyan data bases and existing reports from hospitals in Libya, searches were made for relevant articles about the implementation of Ehealth systems in developing countries. Though there were already assessments made of several countries, none had yet been carried out in Libya. This literature review will give some examples of relevant research discovered during this search and then expand on how these frameworks will be utilised in this assessment on the readiness of Libya for the implementation of Ehealth systems. There was though a limited amount of formal articles on this subject pertaining to developing countries, so a search was made on many databases to find any recent research carried out on assessing the readiness of developing countries for Ehealth implementation.

Blaya et al. (2010) made a review of Ehealth system that had been implemented in developing nations. They found that if a system improved communications between the healthcare institutions, assisted in the management and ordering of medications and helped in monitoring patients that might abandon their care plan, then it could be considered as 'promising'. They found the systems were effective at evaluating personal electronic assistants and mobile apparatus as they improved the collection of data in regards to quality and time taken.

A majority of studies carried out to evaluate Ehealth systems are made once the system has been implemented, as seen in the example of Ammenwerth et al. (2001). Alexander (2007) points out the importance of such studies for evaluating the success of an Ehealth system, though Brender (2006) points out the need for evaluations to take place before the implementation of an Ehealth system in, order to allow decisions to have a better sense of direction. It is the advice of Brender (2006) that the researcher has heeded in the formulation of the research question, tending toward the theory that a readiness evaluation framework is needed before implementing Ehealth systems (Yellowlees 2005; Broens et al. 2007; Khoja et al. 2007a).

Li et al. (2010) cite four main areas to evaluate in a study to assess readiness for implementing an Ehealth system. Those areas are: if it is feasible; does the organisation possess the necessary resources, the risks involved; an assessment needs to be made of what external factors might threaten the project's success, areas where problems may arise; to identify weaknesses in the solution where risks may occur and an assessment of how complete and consistent the solution is.

3 Methods

A mixed method approach was employed for carrying out this research on healthcare institutions, in both rural and urban areas of Libya (Fig. 1) (Molina Azorín and Cameron 2010; Creswell and Plano 2010; Mason 2006; Cathain 2009; Cathain et al. 2008), employing both questionnaires and group interviews. The data from the multi-case study was analysed using the Cresswell framework (2007) (Lynna et al. 2009).

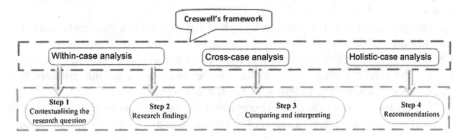

Fig. 1. Cresswell framework (2007), reproduced from (Ahwidy and Pemberton 2016).

Creswell's (2007) description of analysis is that information is broken down into lesser components and reconstituted, forming a larger picture. The research findings will be analysed in this research following Creswell's framework, as shown in Fig. 1.

The formulation of the interview questions and questionnaires was carried out to make sure there was not anything missing by seeing what was needed from the literature review and the Chan framework (2010). The selection of the healthcare institutions was done so that all the major population centres of Libya were covered in five primary areas.

- **Within-case Analysis:** This method for analysing applies to multiple collective or single case studies and the researcher analyses each individual case for themes. While studying multiple cases, researchers can make comparisons within case themes, across multiple cases, in cross case analysis.
- **Cross-case Analysis:** This type of analysis is applicable to collective cases where the researcher is examining more than one case. It entails the examination of themes across cases for discerning themes that are evident in all the cases.
- **Holistic-case Analysis:** This type of data analysis entails the researcher examining the whole case and presenting themes, descriptions and assertions that relate to the entire.

The researcher has chosen to use the three techniques discussed above for analysing data. This is because the study was investigating how much information communication technology was available and being used in each healthcare institution. The data from each healthcare institution will be analysed separately. Ehealth assessments of urban and rural healthcare institutions will also be compared. The data will be analysed in separate categories for rural and urban healthcare institutions. Also data from all the healthcare institutions will be put into a single category for analysis. For the purpose of carrying out the analysis comprehensively, the data will be coded and categorised for all parts of the research. The process for coding and analysing data will be carried out following the suggestions of (Bryman and Burgess 2002) and (Tesch 1990), as follows:

- Create a picture of the whole by reading through the transcript carefully while making notes;
- Go through each document individually, while making sense of its content and make notes in the margins;
- Once this has been carried out for a number of documents, a list should be made of the topics covered. Group similar topics together and make them into columns that can be sorted as leftovers, unique topics and major topics;
- Taking the list, return to the data. Abbreviating the topics as codes, the codes should be written next to the relevant segment of text in order to ascertain if new codes and categories are emerging;
- Come up with wording that best describes each topic and transform them into categories. Make a reduction in the total number of categories by grouping together topics that are related. The interrelationship of categories can be indicated by drawing lines between them;
- Take a decision about what abbreviation will be used for each of the categories and arrange them in alphabetical order;
- Collect together any information that is available from all of the categories and carry out preparatory analysis;

3.1   Research Methods and Sample Size

For the purposes of this study the participants were found in hospitals and clinics within the professions of nursing, hospital administration, ward attendants and doctors. The sample size (see Fig. 2) of this study was 165, with 138 of these returning a questionnaire; as a percentage that worked out at 83.6%. Because 58 of the questionnaires were excluded from the final total because they were filled out incorrectly or superfluous, the final number for analysis was 80 (N = 80).

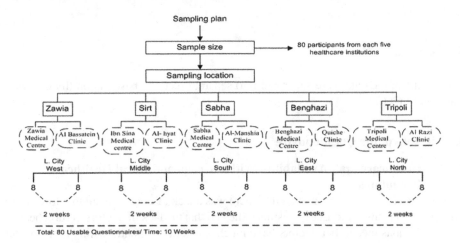

Fig. 2. Sample size, reproduced from (Ahwidy and Pemberton 2016).

The questionnaire was divided into two sections, with one set of questions aimed at general medical staff, the other aimed at administration staff. The questions for the medical staff were designed in order to better understand of the work processes involved in recording the healthcare data of patients, carrying out referrals, consultations and prescriptions. The questions for the administrative staff were formulated in order to better understand of the present ICT infrastructure in the healthcare institutions, the background history of the healthcare institutions and the settings of the healthcare institutions. The formulation of each question was done using the Li et al. (2010) framework for assessing Ehealth readiness. Semi-structured interviews: A total of 40 individual actors (doctors, ward assistants, administrators and nurses) were interviewed in Arabic using semi-structured interview techniques (Table 1). The durations of the interviews varied between 20 and 40 min and averaged out at 30 min for each interview. The total time taken for all the interviews was about 20 h and the details of these interviews are shown below in Table 1.

The reason for interviewing the staff at the healthcare institutions was to find out what their perceptions of Ehealth technologies were and how useful and beneficial they would be if implemented in the healthcare institutions where they worked.

Table 1. Semi-structured interviews, reproduced from (Ahwidy and Pemberton 2016).

Categories of participants	Healthcare institution										
	Tripoli medical centre	Al Razi clinic	Benghazi medical centre	Quiche clinic	Sabha medical centre	Al-Manshia clinic	Ibn Sina medical centre	Al-hyat Clinic	Zawia medical centre	Al-Bassatei n clinic	
Administrators	1	1	1	1	1	1	1	1	1	1	10
Doctors	1	1	1	1	1	1	1	1	1	1	10
Nurses	1	1	1	1	1	1	1	1	1	1	10
Ward assistants	1	1	1	1	1	1	1	1	1		10
Total of participants											40

4   Results

The results of the data were separated into separate sections based upon the Creswell framework (2007).

4.1   Results of the Questionnaire

4.1.1   Healthcare Staff Availability Within Urban and Rural Healthcare Institutions

The results of the research showed that there was a lack of doctors available to work in rural healthcare institutions. The results indicated that the lack of doctors in rural health-care institutions meant that doctors have much less time to spend treating patients and often patients had more severe symptoms as they had further to travel to receive treat-ment and had consequently waited until their condition worsened, whereas patients in urban areas would seek treatment earlier as they lived closer to healthcare institutions and had better transport options available.

4.1.2   ICT Access in Urban and Rural Healthcare Institutions

The study indicated that urban healthcare institutions had more ICT equipment and more reliable internet connections than those in rural areas. The rural healthcare institutions had their internet connections affected by bad phone lines and electrical power supplies that were unreliable. Though the urban healthcare institutions had more computers per doctor than their rural counterparts, this was academic as there were no computers present in the rooms utilised by doctors for their consultations in both rural and urban healthcare institutions, indicating that doctors were not employing computers to carry out consultations. Rather than being used for medical purposes, it was ascertained in the study that the computers in the healthcare institutions were being utilised for adminis-tration purposes. Though the study indicated that rural medical staff were using computers more often than in urban areas, this was only for personal use and was not being carried out during their work time at the healthcare institutions where they worked.

4.2   Results of the Group Interviews

Results of the group interviews were conducted by using qualitative data analysis program called NVIVO (Bazeley 2007; Hamed and Alabri 2013; Ishak and Abu Bakar 2012).

4.2.1   Access to Ehealth Solutions in Urban and Rural Healthcare Institutions

The results of comparing access to Ehealthsolutions, in both rural and urban healthcare institutions, indicated that there were not any Ehealth solutions in any of the healthcare institutions used in the case studies. The participants returned positive feedback regarding the possible future implementation of Ehealth solutions in the healthcare institutions where they worked. It was felt that the implementation of Ehealth technology would improve the recording of patient healthcare records, the treating of patients and the diagnosis of patient's ailments. The results indicated that the participants thought that the use of electronic patient healthcare record systems would greatly improve the service offered to patients and make the job easier for staff and it would stop patients that attended multiple healthcare institutions in order to get repeat prescriptions of medication, therefore stopping fraud occurring and saving the LNHS valuable resources. Presently patient referrals are carried out by giving a patient a handwritten referral on paper to take with them to the healthcare institution to which they have been referred. This meant referral letters were getting lost or patients did not attend. Respondents felt that this task being carried out electronically would eliminate many of these problems.

5   Discussion

5.1   Availability of Medical Staff in Urban and Rural Healthcare Institutions

The issue of physician shortages is far more pressing in rural healthcare institutions than in urban hospitals, though urban clinics do also experience shortages.

The Jennett et al. (2005), Campbell et al. (2001), Blaya and Fraser (2010) indicate that there are many challenges to providing healthcare services in rural areas because of the distances between populations that are dispersed and isolated. Because of these challenges, in rural areas there have often been problems in the recruitment of staff and of them leaving to urban healthcare institutions. In the LNHS, most of the skilled healthcare staff choose to work in urban areas (8280), whereas in rural areas staff are more reluctant to relocate for work (3043) (Hamroush 2014). A lot of rural areas do not have any healthcare staff to provide healthcare to those that require it, so the inhabitants have to travel long distances to seek medical attention, particularly as Libya is so big, yet so sparsely populated.

The lack of healthcare staff in rural healthcare institutions has to be the driving force for attracting more money being invested in Ehealth solutions to help healthcare staff to provide improved healthcare using localised Ehealth frameworks that are appropriate like the framework offered in this research study. Hamroush (2014) compares the availability of physicians in urban and rural healthcare institutions in Libya.

Tables in Hamroush (2014) summarise the average number of physicians that worked in the rural healthcare institutions that were surveyed. The Tables show that on average, there are approximately 73% of physicians in Libya working in urban healthcare institutions, compared to 26% physicians working in rural hospitals. Those percentages indicate there are 20 physicians for every ten thousand local inhabitants in Libya. The following section will focus on how available and accessible ICT technology is within the healthcare institutions chosen for this study.

5.2   The Availability of ICT in Urban and Rural Healthcare Institutions

The study outcomes showed that the availability of ICT and internet connections in both rural and urban healthcare institutions was insufficient for the implementation of Ehealth solutions. In order to function efficiently the ICT systems at each healthcare institution need to be expanded and integrated with other healthcare institutions.

6   Ehealth Maturity Diagram (EMD)

The study outcomes showed that when placed on an Ehealth Maturity Curve (Van de Wetering and Batenburg 2009) the healthcare institutions in both rural and urban areas were at level 0, as can be seen in Fig. 3.

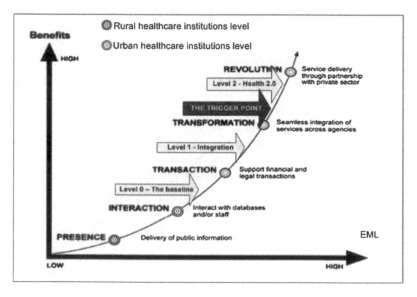

Fig. 3. Phases of Ehealth maturity curve (Van de Wetering and Batenburg 2009), reproduced from (Ahwidy and Pemberton 2016).

Figure 2 above shows that the urban and rural healthcare institutions Ehealth solution levels are at level 0. The healthcare institutions are able to send emails to a central data storage facility for the purpose of administration, but do not appear to use this facility for medical purposes. Despite the existence of some ICT in the healthcare institutions, these systems are not used for contacting other healthcare institutions. This is because of a lack of equipment sometimes or bad internet connections and electrical supplies, but is primarily due to the technophobic attitudes of staff who feel unwilling to embrace new forms of technology (Bain and Rice 2006). Therefore, it is essential if these healthcare institutions are to rise above level 0, a Provincial Ehealth framework be formulated using these findings to facilitate a plan for the future in order for the healthcare institutions to move to level 2 on the Ehealth maturity curve. Because of this the Provincial Ehealth framework was formulated, as can be seen below in Fig. 4.

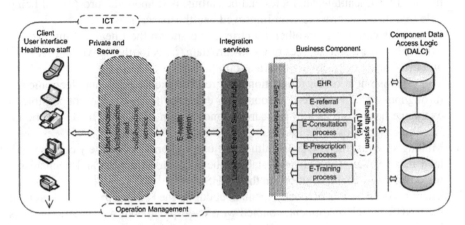

Fig. 4. Provincial Ehealth framework, reproduced from (Ahwidy and Pemberton 2016).

The Provincial Ehealth framework architecture highlights the need for the services offered in the healthcare institutions to be integrated online by using an Ehealth service hub that supports the whole of the LNHS and for data to be stored electronically rather than by using paper records as at present.

7   Strategy for Ehealth in the LNHS

In order for the LNHS to raise its maturity levels for the implementation of Ehealth technology, it needs to persuade LNHS staff and patients to adopt Ehealth technologies. This can be carried out at a local level throughout the LNHS, though this will need to be orchestrated at a national level through training, education and programmesto encourage compliance and providing incentives.

The drive to raise the maturity levels for the implementation of Ehealth technology throughout the LNHS needs to focus in several areas. This is a non exhaustive list of some of those:

1. LNHS users need to be made aware of what is available to them through use of Ehealth in the LNHS through media and other sources and be shown the advantages of accessing their individual healthcare records. Public support for Ehealth

developments will encourage politicians to invest in developing ICTinfrastructures and to ensure that broadband speeds are sufficient and telephone connections are reliable.

2. Healthcare institutions need to be given financial aid with implementing Ehealth systems to encourage their widespread usage. There needs to be a direct link between usage of Ehealth technology and funding.

3. It is of great importance for a healthcare system utilising Ehealth technologies to ensure that sufficient numbers of healthcare staff have been trained to high enough standards to operate the technology effectively. Staff also need to be convinced of the need for Ehealth technologies and be enthusiastic about the prospect of being able to utilise it in order to offer improved healthcare services.

4. Researches carried out in other countries have shown the Ehealth solutions that need to be prioritised: sources of healthcare data, tools for the delivery of services and the sharing of electronic information.

5. The establishment of the foundation required for exchanging data electronically throughout the LNHS. This development is essential because if it is not possible to exchange healthcare data in a secure manner within the LNHS there will be no Ehealth capabilities in the LNHS.

6. Making sure that the LNHS Ehealth adoption program is effectively coordinated, lead and overseen. This will help establish the necessary structures and mechanisms for governing Ehealth solutions in the LNHS.

7. There needs to be a lot of money spent on updating the IT infrastructure throughout the LNHS as lack investment, coupled with widespread civil war and looting, has left the LNHS in short supply of basic computer equipment.

8. Ehealth information stored by the LNHS needs to be standardised throughout the LNHS in order that information can be exchanged effectively. This can be carried out through central planning establishing implementation procedures along with Ehealth implementation.

9. It is essential that the LNHS protects sensitive healthcare data so that it remains private. In order for this to succeed there needs to be a robust and secure security system implemented throughout the LNHS.

10. Healthcare information requires a regime for identifying and authenticating information as quickly as the LNHS can manage so that it can be accessed and shared securely.

11. Facilitating healthcare institutions in the establishment of ICT that are appropriate for their individual needs.

12. Coordinating healthcare institutions to create ICT infrastructures that are sustainable.

13. Supporting healthcare institutions to connect to a nationwide fibre optic network for sharing data and connecting to other healthcare institutions.

14. Implementing policies for the exchange of information between healthcare institutions that do not contravene any privacy laws.

15. Implementing E-learning for improving education levels.

16. The construction of the Ehealth capabilities of the LNHS incrementally and prag-
matically, while initially investing in Ehealth technologies that will afford the most
benefits to users of the LNHS.
17. Provide help to those areas of the LNHS that require it, but not at the expensive of
those that would like to develop at a faster pace.
18. Creating processes for EHRs, E-consultations, E-prescriptions, E-referrals and E-
training systems.

8 The Study's Limitations

The largest challenge in carrying out this case study for the researcher was not just the
large distances between healthcare institutions that were travelled, in order to create as
balanced a reflection as possible of opinions in the LNHS, but the state of warfare that
existed in the country at the time between rival tribal factions.

The other limitation in this study is that the framework has not been used in practice
to see where it does not work, so that it can be improved. This is because it would require
a lot of money to test it that is not currently available in Libya, though when the
researcher presented his findings to experts in Libya it was received positively.

A lot of the limitations inherent in the research technique and methodology have
already been covered in the writings above. Further factors affecting the efficiency of
the research were the time limitations imposed by the LNHS and the Libyan culture
itself. The reason for employing the methods of questionnaire and interview in this study
was to enhance the level of confidentiality that the participants would enjoy. That a high
level of privacy was maintained was of utmost importance. Another hurdle placed in
the researcher's way in carrying out the interviews was that of gender. Because of the
restrictions within Libyan culture regarding the mixing of males and females, the
researcher being male needed to employ females to carry out such tasks. It was expected
that by placing guarantees of anonymity the participants would therefore feel more
relaxed and deliver answers that were more accurate, confidential and honest. Time
presented a serious limitation to the researcher due to healthcare institutions allowing
interviews to be for no longer than 25 min. This was because the LNHS authorities did
not want the medical staff's private time intruded upon, hence limiting interview time
to that reserved for giving lectures, thus placing a limitation upon the quantity of variables that could be harvested.

The fact that the participant's confidential details were self reported creates yet
another limitation to the study. This is because it may create inaccuracies, thus information that is technologically, socially, culturally or medically influenced, may need to
be considered as differing somewhat to reality when medical ISs are being planned.

9 Suggested Solutions for Overcoming Barriers for the LNHS

A challenge for healthcare institutions in the LNHS with the introduction of Ehealth
technologies would be a serious lack in experienced healthcare staff. In order to alleviate
this deficiency the LNHS needs to formulate a menu of training courses available for

staff, so that whichever Ehealth systems are going to be installed in a healthcare institution, then the healthcare staff receive the appropriate courses.

To educate staff that have absolutely no experience in operating Ehealth equipment is an enormous challenge, especially as so few have experience in even using computers for personal use as in the LNHS. The thoroughness of such training though would greatly influence the success rates that can expected from the implementation of Ehealth technology in a healthcare institution. It is also very important that the training program be aligned with the views of the director of the Ehealth implementation, particularly when that person has been brought in to that environment for the purpose of directing it. In order to command loyalty from existing staff it could be very beneficial to incorporate a leader in the community that commands a lot of respect to assist in the planning stage of the project so that healthcare staff and local residents feel some loyalty and inclusion in the project.

The leader in the community that would be incorporated might be someone who had been mayor or an important business leader, though it is a good idea to make sure that they were a popular mayor or not a business leader who had closed down many work places or been suspected of corruption. This person could then be the chair person for a committee that drafts possible outcomes for the project. It is also prudent to include in this committee someone who previously presided over the transition of a healthcare institution to Ehealth technologies. They could then provide advice to the chair person who has the respect of staff and community alike. The consultant would also provide assistance in choosing an experienced program director to take over the project once it begins to take place.

Once the planning stage is completed and the project commences, the appointment of the program director is a very important move. They need to be skilled in many areas and be able to handle public speaking while communicating to the public the progress and visions of the project as well as managing many departments in the implementation of Ehealth technologies.

It is a good idea for the LNHS to garner support within local communities for the transition to Ehealth technologies prior to appointment of a program director. The director will then have an easier time in convincing locals in rural areas of the advantages of accessing healthcare via E-consultations rather than travelling long distances for consultations.

It is also a wise decision to include a well respected member of the local community in the planning committee, as their inclusion can influence the levels of acceptance and participation that greet such programs as E-learning projects. If a community is enthusiastic about an Ehealth implementation, then the chance are that more will enrol to train for a career in healthcare locally. A selection of community leaders could be invited to attend conference that last two or three days where a selection of leaders in the healthcare industry attend and educate these people on the intricacies of their professions and explain the potentials of Ehealth technologies. This has been tried in developed countries where it has had great success, though in the view of the researcher this might be even more successful in Libya, as there is great respect held for community leaders there (Sunyaev 2011).

The work entailed in gaining the support of communities may be time consuming and expensive, but ultimately brings many rewards such as the support of politicians, who not only feel great admiration for high tech developments that benefit the public, but if the public associate them with such developments their popularity may rise among voters.

A key factor in any development within the healthcare sector is monitoring and evaluating (M&E). M&E will help those managing such projects in assessing if they are on course for their objective, or if they need to direct the project in a different direction. Using a solid M&E strategy for the implementation of Ehealth services would help the MOH to upgrade services in the LNHS more effectively and efficiently. Utilising the M&E approach would mean that it could be seen whether or not the MOH was following the plan for the implementation of Ehealth services efficiently.

For the implementation of Ehealth technologies within the LNHS it is imperative that there be adequate trained healthcare staff available. This would involve getting staff to train in specific skills so that all Ehealth technologies implemented will be operated competently. This would entail the creation of an Ehealth competency framework for healthcare staff, so that each task that is required for the system to operate efficiently, has adequate healthcare staff trained to a required standard.

The users of the LNHS need to be confident that their personal healthcare data will remain confidential if an EHR system is implemented in the LNHS. In order to do this the Libyan government would need to implement legislation that would ensure the protection of personal data of patients in the LNHS.

In many countries governments have been slow to legislate to protect the privacy rights of patients private data when entered into Ehealth systems. Patients often have no rights should their data be accessed without their consent. It is imperative that if in Libya Ehealth systems are implemented, then legislation should be passed to protect patient's personal healthcare data.

The LNHS needs to develop guidelines for healthcare leaders for the implementation of Ehealth. This should include the 'sharing of a vision' about beginning a program, setting up goals for the program to achieve, the sharing of resources and risk sharing and how to create work environments that are beneficial to staff and patients alike.

10   Conclusions

After exploring the Ehealth readiness assessment models that were currently used in both developing and developed nations, and assessing the five urban and rural healthcare institutions chosen for Ehealth readiness in LNHS and analysing the research findings, the researcher will now set out the reached conclusions of research study, namely that: when the findings of the survey for rural and urban healthcare institutions were comparatively analysed and interpreted through use of the Ehealth maturity curve, it showed that urban healthcare institutions were at the interaction stage and rural healthcare institutions were at the presence stage. Both stages though are level zero. These results were utilised for making the recommendations that were shown above and were utilised for compiling the Ehealth framework that has been compiled for the LNHS. The research findings also showed that rural hospitals and urban clinics do not have enough doctors, hence they are overworked; Ehealth could allow rural healthcare staff to contact urban doctors for advice; rural healthcare institutions need Ehealth to make up for lack of staff. The researcher also recommended that, for successful adaptation of Ehealth technology into the Libyan National Healthcare Services, the Ehealth systems need to be made interoperable so that different systems and information sources are brought together into more powerful integrated systems; and the Ehealth system will help healthcare staff in healthcare institutions in the creation, maintenance and sharing of electronic patient health records. To conclude, this research study has laid out areas that require attention in order for the LNHS to implement successful Ehealth technologies. For each area there have been strategic objectives recorded, that should be followed in order to lead the LNHS to move from level 0 on the Ehealth maturity curve to a level 2, hence providing the necessary patient data that is needed when treating patients (electronic patient health records), enhancing the surveillance and monitoring of activities, reducing errors in the prescription of medication.

References

Ahwidy, M., Pemberton, L.: What changes need to be made within the LNHS for ehealth systems to be successfully implemented? In: Proceedings of the International Conference on Information and Communication Technologies for Ageing Well and e-Health, pp. 71–79 (2016). doi:10.5220/0005620400710079, ISBN 978-989-758-180-9

Ammenwerth, E., Eichstadter, R., Haux, R., Pohl, U., Rebel, S., Ziegler, S.: A randomized evaluation of a computer-based nursing documentation system. Methods Inf. Med. **40**, 61–68 (2001)

Alexander, H.: Health-service evaluations: should we expect the results to change practice? Evaluation **9**(4), 405–414 (2007)

Bain, C.D., Rice, M.L.: The influence of gender on attitudes, perception, and use of technology. J. Res. Technol. Educ. **39**(2), 119–132 (2006)

Bazeley, P.: Qualitative Data Analysis with NVivo, pp. 6–15. Sage Publications Ltd, London (2007)

Bilbey, N., Lalani, S.: Canadian health care: a focus on rural medicine. UBCMJ **2**(2), 7–8 (2013). aVancouver Fraser Medical Program 2013, UBC Faculty of Medicine, Vancouver, BC

Blaya, J., Fraser, H.F.: Implementing medical information systems in developing countries, what works and what doesn't. In: AMIA 2010 Symposium Proceedings, p. 232 (2010)

Brender, J.: Evaluation Methods for Health Informatics. Elsevier Inc., London (2006)

Bryman, A., Burgess, R.G.: Analyzing Qualitative Data. The Taylor and Francis e-Library, London and New York (2002)

Broens, T., Huis in't Veld, R.M.H.A., Vollenbroek-Hutten, M.M.R., Hermens, H.J., Van Halteren, A.T., Niewenhuis, L.J.M.: Determinants of successful telemedicine implementations. J. Telemed. Telecare **6**(13), 303–309 (2007)

Cathain, A.: Mixed methods research in the health sciences: a quiet revolution. J. Mixed Methods Res. **3**, 3–6 (2009)

Cathain, A., Murphy, E., Nicholl, J.: The quality of mixed methods studies in health services research. J. Health Serv. Res. Policy **13**(2), 92–98 (2008). The Royal Society of Medicine Press Ltd.

Campbell, J.D., Harris, K.D., Hodge, R.: Introducing telemedicine technology to rural physicians and settings. J. Fam. Pract. **50**, 419–424 (2001)

Creswell, J.W.: Qualitative Inquiry and Research Design: Choosing Among Five Approaches, 2nd edn. Sage Publications, Inc., Thousand Oaks (2007)

Creswell, J., Plano Clark, V.: Designing and Conducting Mixed Methods Research, 2nd edn. Sage, Thousand Oaks (2010)

Chan, C.V., Kaufman, D.R.: A technology selection framework for supporting delivery of patient-oriented health interventions in developing countries. J. Biomed. Inform. **43**, 300–306 (2010)

Hamed, H., Alabri, S.: Using NVIVO for data analysis in qualitative research. Int. Interdiscip. J. Educ. **2**(2), 181–186 (2013). Ministry of Education, Sultanate of Oman

Hamroush, F.: Medical Studies & Training: Challenges and Opportunities. Minister of Health in the Transitional Libyan Government, Libya Higher Education Forum 2014, London (2014)

Hossein, S.M.: Consideration the relationship between ICT and Ehealth. J. Biol. Agricult. Healthc. **2**(8), 49–59 (2012). International Institute for Science, Technology & Education

Ishak, N.M., Abu Bakar, A.Y.: Qualitative data management and analysis using NVivo: an approach used to examine leadership qualities among student leaders. Educ. Res. J. **2**(3), 94–103 (2012). Int. Res. J.

Jennett, P., Yeo, M., Pauls, M., Graham, J.: Organizational readiness for telemedicine: implications for success and failure. J. Telemed. Telecare **9**(Suppl 2), S27–S30 (2004)

Jennett, P., Jackson, A., Ho, K., Healy, T., Kazanjian, A., Woollard, R., et al.: The essence of telehealth readiness in rural communities: an organizational perspective. Telemed. J. Ehealth **11**, 137–145 (2005)

Khoja, S., Scott, R., Ishaq, A., Mohsin, M.: Testing reliability of ehealth readiness assessment tools for developing countries. Ehealth Int. J. **3**(1), 425–431 (2007a)

Khoja, S., Scott, R., Casebeer, A., Mohsin, M., Ishaq, A., Gilani, S.: e-Health readiness assessment tools for healthcare institutions in developing countries. Telemed. eHealth **13**(4), 425–432 (2007b)

Kwankam, S.: What e-Health can offer? Bull. World Health Organ. **82**(10), 800–802 (2004)

Lau, F., Price, M., Keshavjee, K.: From benefit evaluation to clinical adoption: making sense of health information system success in Canada. Electron. Healthc. **9**(4), 39–45 (2011)

Li, J.: E-health readiness framework from electronic health records perspective. Australia (2010)

Ludwick, A., Doucette, J.: Adopting electronic medical records in primary care lessons learned from health information systems implementation experience in seven countries. Int. J. Med. Inform. **78**, 22–31 (2009)

Lynna, J., Martens, J., Washington, E., Steele, D., Washburn, E.: A cross case analysis of gender issues in desktop virtual reality learning environment. J. Ind. Teacher Educ. **46**(3), 51–89 (2009). Oklahoma State University

Mason, J.: Mixing methods in a qualitatively driven way. Qual. Res. **6**, 9–25 (2006)

Molina Azorín, J., Cameron, R.: The application of mixed methods in organisational research: a literature review. Electron. J. Bus. Res. Methods **8**(2), 95–105 (2010)

Sunyaev, A.: Health-Care Telematics in Germany: Design and Application of a Security Analysis Method. Springer, Germany (2011)

Tesch, R.: Qualitative Research: Analysis Types and Software Tools. Falmer, New York (1990)

Van de Wetering, R., Batenburg, R.: A PACS maturity model: a systematic meta analytic review on maturation and evolvability of PACS in the hospital enterprise. Int. J. Med. Inform. **78**, 127–140 (2009)

Yellowlees, P.: Successfully developing a telemedicine system. J. Telemed. Telecare **11**(7), 331–336 (2005)

Wong, L.P.: Data analysis in qualitative research: a brief guide to using Nvivo. Malays. Fam. Phys. **3**(1), 14–20 (2008)

Improving Human Motion Identification Using Motion Dependent Classification

Evangelia Pippa[1]($\boxtimes$), Iosif Mporas[2],
and Vasileios Megalooikonomou[1]

[1] Multidimentional Data Analysis and Knowledge Discovery Laboratory,
Department of Computer Engineering and Informatics,
University of Patras, Rion-Patras, Greece
{pippa, vasilis}@ceid.upatras.gr
[2] School of Engineering and Technology,
University of Hertfordshire, Hatfield, UK
i.mporas@herts.ac.uk

Abstract. In this article, we present a new methodology for human motion identification based on motion dependent binary classifiers that afterwards fuse their decisions to identify an Activity of Daily Living (ADL). Temporal and spectral features extracted from the sensor signals (accelerometer and gyroscope) and concatenated to a single feature vector are used to train motion dependent binary classification models. Each individual model is capable to recognize one motion versus all the others. Afterwards the decisions are combined by a fusion function using as weights the sensitivity values derived from the evaluation of each motion dependent classifier on the provided training set. The proposed methodology was evaluated using SVMs for the motion dependent classifiers and is compared against the common multiclass classification approach optimized using either feature selection or subject dependent classification. The classification accuracy of the proposed methodology reaches 99% offering competitive performance comparing to the other approaches.

Keywords: Human motion identification · ADLs · Classification · Fusion · Feature extraction · Accelerometers · Gyroscopes

1 Introduction

The ageing population around the world is increasing and it is estimated that two billion people will be aged over 65 years by 2050. This will affect the planning and delivery of health and social care as well as the clinical condition of frailty. Frailty is a medical syndrome which is characterized by diminished strength, endurance, and reduced physiologic function that increases an individual's vulnerability for developing increased dependency and/or death [1]. Frailty is characterized by multiple pathologies such as weight loss, weakness, low activity, slow motor performance, balance and gait abnormalities, as well as cognitive ones [2]. Frailty increases risks of incident falls, worsening of mobility, disability, hospitalization or institutionalization, and mortality [3–5], which in turn increase the burden to cares and costs to the society.

© Springer International Publishing AG 2017
C. Röcker et al. (Eds.): ICT4AWE 2016, CCIS 736, pp. 49–65, 2017.
DOI: 10.1007/978-3-319-62704-5_4

It is assumed that early intervention with frail persons will improve quality of life and reduce health services costs. Thus, it is essential to develop real life tools for the assessment of physiologic reserve and the need to test interventions that alter the natural course of frailty since frailty is a dynamic and not an irreversible process. Several efforts have been done in this direction through research and development activities. In [6] an Ecosystem for training, informing and providing tools, processes, methodologies for ICT and active, healthy aging was developed mainly targeting to caregivers, older people and general population. In [7] an interactive tabletop platform able to integrate potentialities derived from both technology and leisure activities was designed. Another purpose of [7] was the monitoring of the older people status, with information about his/her progression/regression in cognitive health. In [8] a home-care solution that will address older people living in the community in a preventive manner and rely on ICT and virtual reality gaming through the exploitation of haptic technologies, vision control and context awareness methods was developed and integrated, while promising to redefine fall prevention by motivating people to be more active, in a friendly way and with tele-supervision if necessary. In [9] a more holistic, personalized, medically efficient and economical monitoring system for people with epilepsy was provided. In [10] multidisciplinary research areas in serious games, social networking, wireless sensor networks, activity recognition and contextualization, behavioral pattern analysis were combined in pilot setups involving both older users and care providers. In [11] a mobile, personalized assistant for older people was developed, using cutting edge technologies such as advanced speech interaction, which helps them stay independent, coordinate with careers and foster their social contacts. In [12] new, economically sustainable home assistance service which extends older people independent living was introduced, measuring the impact of monitoring, cognitive training and e-Inclusion services on the quality of life of older people, on the cost of social and healthcare delivered to them, and on a number of social indicators. In [13] the objective was to develop and test a proactive personal robotic, integrated with innovative sensors, localization and communication technologies, and smart textiles to support independent living for older adults, in their home or in various degrees of institutionalization, with a focus on health, nutrition, well-being, and safety. In [14] innovative ICT-based solutions for the detection of falls in ageing people were studied, covering prevention and detection of falls in different circumstances.

Human motion monitoring is a must in surveillance of older people, since the related information is crucial for understanding the physical status and the behavior of the older people. Older people suffering from frailty are often required to fulfill a program of activity which follows a training schedule that is integrated within their daily activities [15]. Therefore, the detection of activities such as walking or walking-upstairs becomes quite useful to provide valuable information to the caregiver about the patient's behavior. Under conditions of daily living, human-activity recognition could be performed using objective and reliable techniques.

Monitoring the activities of daily living requires non-intrusive technology. The main devices an older person can be instrumented through are classified into two main categories based on the used technology: vision-based and wearable. In computer vision, complex sensors such as cameras that continuously record the movement of the elderly have been used to submit the acquired data to specific image algorithms that recognize human activities. In general, tracking and activity recognition using computer vision-based techniques perform quite well in a laboratory conditions or at well-controlled environments. However, their accuracy is lower in real-home settings, due to the high-level activities that take place in the natural environments, as well as the variable lighting or clutter [16]. Furthermore, computer vision methods require a pre-built infrastructure which instead of the time and cost of installation introduce limitations for the space of application since it is hard to be used outdoors. As a result, wearable devices such as body-attached accelerometers and gyroscopes are commonly used as an alternative in order to assess variable daily living activities. The human motion detection problem using wearable sensors is an emerging area of research due to their low-power requirements, small size, non-intrusiveness and ability to provide data regarding human motion. The acquired data can be processed using signal processing and pattern recognition methods, in order to obtain nearly accurate recognition of human motion.

Data acquired from wearable sensors have been used to evaluate several human-activity recognition methods proposed in the literature. Acceleration signals have been used to analyze and classify different kinds of activity [16, 17] or applied for recognizing a wide set of daily physical activities [18]. Feature selection techniques have also been investigated [19]. The reclassification step introduced by Bernecker et al. [20] has been demonstrated to increase motion recognition accuracy. The results achieved by the on-board processing technique for the real-time classification system proposed by Karantonis et al. [21] demonstrate the feasibility of implementing an accelerometer-based, real-time movement classifier using embedded intelligence. Khan et al. [16] proposed a system that uses a hierarchical-recognition scheme, i.e. the state recognition at the lower level using statistical features and the activity recognition at the upper level using the augmented feature vector followed by linear discriminant analysis. Considering the machine learning algorithms for human motion identification that are found in the literature, the most widely used are artificial neural networks [21–23], Naive-Bayes [18] and support vector machines [19, 24–26].

In this article we focus on the physiological function and motor performance thus we present a human motion identification scheme together with preliminary evaluation results, which will be further exploited within the FrailSafe [27] project architecture. The proposed scheme uses temporal and spectral features extracted from the sensor signals and concatenated to a single feature vector to train motion dependent binary classification models that afterwards fuse their decisions to identify ADLs. This scheme is compared against the common multiclass classification scheme after its optimization using two different strategies.

The reminder of this article is organized as follows. In Sect. 2 we present the FrailSafe concept. In Sect. 3 we describe the proposed human motion identification scheme and the common multiclass approach with respect to the optimization strategies. In Sects. 4 and 5 we present the experimental setup and the evaluation results respectively. Finally, in Sect. 6 we conclude this work.

2 The FrailSafe Concept

FrailSafe aims to better understand frailty and its relation to co-morbidities, to develop quantitative and qualitative measures to define frailty and to use these measures to predict short and long-term outcome. In order to achieve these goals real life tools for the assessment of physiological reserve and of external challenges will be developed. These tools will provide an adaptive model (sensitive to changes) in order that pharmaceutical and non-pharmaceutical interventions, which will be designed to delay, arrest or even reverse the transition to frailty. Moreover, FrailSafe targets at creating "prevent-frailty" evidence based recommendations for older people regarding activities of daily living, lifestyle and nutrition, as well as strengthening the motor cognitive, and other "anti-frailty" activities through the delivery of personalized treatment programs, monitoring alerts, guidance and education. The FrailSafe conceptual diagram for motion monitoring is illustrated in Fig. 1.

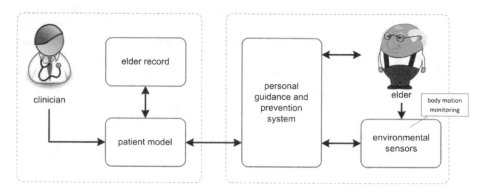

Fig. 1. The FrailSafe conceptual diagram for motion monitoring reproduced from [28].

Through patient-specific interventions, FrailSafe aims to define a frailty measure. This measure is initially constructed from prior knowledge on the field, and then globally updated based on analysis of long-term observations of all older peoples' states. This update is then applied to the individual patient models, modifying them accordingly, to fit different needs per patient. The monitoring of the older people's motion activity is performed through the environmental sensors module, which includes accelerometer sensors for the monitoring of the human motions. Details about the motion identification implementation are provided in the next section.

3 Methodology for Human Motion Identification

3.1 Motion Dependent Classification Scheme

The presented methodology for human motion identification will be used as part of an end-to-end system for sensing and predicting risk of frailty taking into account associated co-morbidities using advanced personalized models as well as delaying frailty using advanced interventions.

The proposed classification methodology can be used as a core module in order to discriminate the detected motions to six basic activities: walking, walking-upstairs, walking-downstairs, sitting, standing and laying. The block diagram of the overall workflow for learning the activity classifiers is illustrated in Fig. 2.

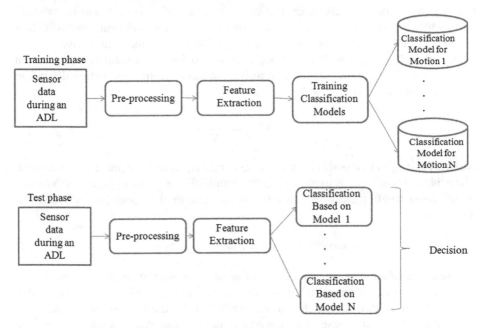

Fig. 2. Motion Dependent Classification of ADLs.

The multi-parametric sensor (accelerometer and gyroscope) data are pre-processed as in [24–26] by applying noise filters and then sampled in fixed-width sliding windows $W_i, 1 \leq i \leq I$ (frames) of 2.56 s and 50% overlap. The sensor acceleration signal, which has gravitational and body motion components, was separated using a Butterworth low-pass filter into body acceleration and gravity. From each frame, a vector of features $V_i \in R^k, k = |F_T| + |F_F|$ was obtained by calculating variables from the time $F_T^i \in R^{|F_T|}$ and frequency domain $F_F^i \in R^{|F_F|}$.

The extracted time domain and frequency domain features are concatenated into a single feature vector as a representative signature for each frame. Details on the type of extracted features are provided in Sect. 4.

All frames are used as input to the human motion identification module which classifies basic activities of daily living (ADLs) in order to obtain some preliminary evaluation results for the proposed scheme. In this module, N motion dependent binary classification models that have been built in the training phase, are used to label the frames. N is the number of the discrete motions/classes; here $N = 6$ since the motions to be identified include six ADLs: walking, walking-upstairs, walking-downstairs, sitting, standing and laying. Each classification model is trained as a binary model capable to discriminate each motion from all the others, e.g. the first classification model performs walking vs. all remaining ADLs classification, the second classification model performs walking-upstairs vs. all remaining ADLs classification, etc.

During the training phase of the classification scheme, frames with known class labels (manually labeled) are used to train the N classification models. For this purpose, the same training set is labeled with N different ways to obtain N motion dependent binary classification models. Each time the examined motion is treated as the positive class while a negative class label is assigned to all of the remaining motions. In a further step, in order to obtain appropriate weights to fuse the individual classifiers, we evaluated each of the classification models using a 10-fold cross-validation protocol on the corresponding training sets. The sensitivity achieved from each motion dependent classification model $(S_i, 1 < i < N)$ and defined as:

$$S_i = \frac{TP_i}{TP_i + FN_i}.$$ (1)

where TP_i denotes true positives of classifier i and FN_i its false negatives, is calculated. The achieved sensitivity is used as a weight to multiply the decision $(d_i, 1 < i < N)$ taken by the corresponding classifier i in a fusion function used to combine the individual decisions:

$$Decision = S_1d_1 + S_2d_2 + \ldots + S_Nd_N.$$ (2)

Here, we selected sensitivity instead of another measure such as accuracy since a measure of the proportion of the positives (i.e., the motion under consideration) that were correctly identified as such is more appropriate for the purpose of fusion.

During the test phase the unknown multi-parametric sensor signals are pre-processed and parameterized with similar setup as in the training phase. Each extracted feature vector is provided as input to each one of the N trained motion dependent classification models. Each of them takes a binary decision $(d_i, 1 < i < N)$. Finally, the N individual decisions are combined using the fusion function of Eq. (2).

3.2 Multiclass Classification Scheme

The proposed scheme is compared to the common multiclass classification scheme, which is widely used in such applications. The block diagram of the workflow for learning the multiclass classifier of this scheme is illustrated in Fig. 3.

In order to make a fair comparison, the multi-parametric sensor (accelerometer and gyroscope) data are pre-processed and parameterized with the same features as in the motion dependent classification scheme. Once again, the extracted time domain and frequency domain features are concatenated to a single feature vector as a representative signature for each frame. However, in this scheme all frames are used as input to the human motion identification module which directly classifies the N basic activities of daily living (ADLs). In this module, a model for multiclass classification between

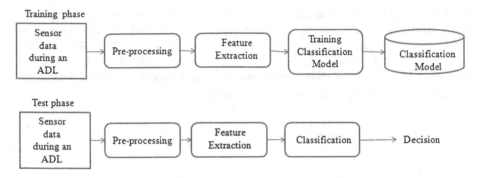

Fig. 3. Multiclass classification scheme reproduced from [28].

N (here $N = 6$) basic ADLs (walking, walking-upstairs, walking-downstairs, sitting, standing and laying), which has been previously built in a training phase, is used to label the frames. Each frame is classified independently.

During the training phase of the classification architecture, frames with known class labels (labeled manually) are used to train the multiclass classification model. During the test phase the unknown multi-parametric sensor signals are pre-processed and parameterized with similar setup as in the training phase. Each extracted feature vector is provided as input to the trained classifier.

In a further, step we attempt to optimize the multiclass classification scheme following two different strategies. On the one hand, we perform feature selection by feature ranking prior to classification while on the other hand we perform subject dependent classification.

Feature Selection. Regarding the first optimization strategy, we examined the discriminative ability of the extracted features for the human motion identification [28]. The ReliefF algorithm [29] (which is an extension of an earlier algorithm called Relief [30]) was used for estimating the importance of each feature in multiclass classification. In the ReliefF algorithm the weight of any given feature decreases if the squared Euclidean distance of that feature to nearby instances of the same class is more than the distance to nearby instances of the other class. ReliefF is considered one of the most successful feature ranking algorithms due to its simplicity and effectiveness [31–33] (only linear time in the number of given features and training samples is required), noise tolerance and robustness in detecting relevant features effectively, even when these features are highly dependent on other features [31, 34]. Furthermore, ReliefF avoids any exhaustive or heuristic search compared with conventional wrapper methods and usually performs better compared to filter methods due to the performance feedback of a nonlinear classifier when searching for useful features [32].

The performance of the method, in terms of accuracy for different number of N-best features (N = 10, 20, 30,... 560), with respect to the ReliefF feature ranking algorithm was examined. The subset that achieved the highest classification accuracy was selected and used to optimize the performance of the multiclass classification scheme.

Subject Dependent Classification. Regarding the second optimization strategy, we simply trained a subject specific multiclass classification model for each subject separately instead of one global model trained on several subjects [28]. This strategy makes the classification procedure an easier task since inter-subject variability does not affect the accuracy of the model. However, such an approach has the serious disadvantage of requiring training data from each subject.

4 Experimental Setup

4.1 Dataset

The previously described classification methodology was evaluated on multi-parametric data from the UCI HAR Dataset [24]. The dataset consists of accelerometer and gyroscope recordings from 30 volunteers within an age bracket of 19-48 years when performing six activities (walking, walking-upstairs, walking-downstairs sitting, standing, laying). For the experiments each person worn a smartphone (Samsung Galaxy S II) on the waist. Using its embedded accelerometer and gyroscope, 3-axial linear acceleration and 3-axial angular velocity at a constant rate of 50 Hz were captured. The data were labeled manually using the corresponding video recordings which were captured during the experiments.

4.2 Feature Extraction and Classification Algorithm

Initially, the sensor signals (accelerometer and gyroscope) were pre-processed as proposed in [24–26] in order to proceed with feature extraction. The features selected for this analysis are those proposed in [24–26], which come from the accelerometer and gyroscope 3-axial raw signals denoted as tAcc-XYZ and tGyro-XYZ with prefix 't' used to denote time. The sampling frequency of these time domain signals was 50 Hz. In order to remove noise Anguita et al. performed low pass filtering using a median filter and a 3rd order low pass Butterworth filter with a corner frequency of 20 Hz. Then, in order to separate the acceleration signal into body and gravity acceleration signals denoted as tBodyAcc-XYZ and tGravityAcc-XYZ, they used another low pass Butterworth filter with a corner frequency of 0.3 Hz.

Subsequently, Jerk signals denoted as tBodyAccJerk-XYZ and tBodyGyroJerk-XYZ were obtained by the time derivation of the body linear acceleration and angular velocity. Also they used the Euclidean norm to calculate the magnitude of these three-dimensional signals yielding the following signals: tBodyAccMag, tGravityAccMag, tBodyAccJerk Mag, tBodyGyroMag and tBodyGyroJerkMag.

Finally, a Fast Fourier Transform (FFT) was applied to signals tBodyAcc-XYZ, tBodyAccJerk-XYZ, tBodyGyro-XYZ, tBodyAccJerkMag, tBodyGyroMag, tBody-GyroJerkMag producing fBodyAcc-XYZ, fBodyAccJerk-XYZ, fBodyGyro-XYZ, fBodyAccJerkMag, fBodyGyroMag, fBodyGyroJerkMag. Here, the prefix 'f' was used to indicate frequency domain signals.

These signals were used to estimate variables of the feature vector for each pattern: '-XYZ' is used to denote 3-axial signals in the X, Y and Z directions. The aforementioned signals which were produced by processing accordingly the initial sensor recordings are tabulated in Table 1.

Table 1. Pre-processed Signals reproduced from [28].

Signals
tBodyAcc-XYZ
tGravityAcc-XYZ
tBodyAccJerk-XYZ
tBodyGyro-XYZ
tBodyGyroJerk-XYZ
tBodyAccMag
tGravityAccMag
tBodyAccJerkMag
tBodyGyroMag
tBodyGyroJerkMag
fBodyAcc-XYZ
fBodyAccJerk-XYZ
fBodyGyro-XYZ
fBodyAccMag
fBodyAccJerkMag
fBodyGyroMag
fBodyGyroJerkMag

The set of features that were extracted from these signals are those proposed by Anguita et al. including the mean value, the standard deviation, the median absolute deviation, the largest value in array, the smallest value in array, the signal magnitude area, the energy measure as the sum of the squares divided by the number of values, the interquartile range, the signal entropy, the autoregresesion coefficients with Burg order equal to 4, the correlation coefficient between two signal, the index of the frequency component with largest magnitude, the weighted average of the frequency components to obtain a mean frequency, the skewness of the frequency domain signal, the kurtosis of the frequency domain signal, the energy of a frequency interval within the 64 bins of the FFT of each window and the angle between two vectors.

Additional vectors were obtained by averaging the signals in a signal window sample. These are used on the angle variable (see Table 2). In conclusion, for each record a 561-feature vector with the aforementioned time and frequency domain variables was provided.

The computed feature vectors were used to train either six binary classification models (walking-vs-all remaining, walking-upstairs-vs-all remaining, walking-downstairs-vs-all remaining, sitting-vs-all remaining, standing-vs-all remaining, and laying-vs-all remaining) for the motion dependent classification scheme or a multiclass classification

Table 2. Additional Signals reproduced from [28].

Additional siganls
gravityMean
tBodyAccMean
tBodyAccJerkMean
tBodyGyroMean
tBodyGyroJerkMean

model for the multiclass classification scheme. In the last case, the multiclass classification model is trained on the reduced feature vector obtained by feature selection for the first optimization strategy or on the subject specific data for the second optimization strategy. In order to evaluate the ability of the extracted features to discriminate between ADLs we examined the SMO [35, 36] with RBF kernel classification algorithm, which was implemented by the WEKA machine learning toolkit [37]. SMO algorithm is an implementation of Support Vector Machines provided by the WEKA toolkit. Here we selected SMO for the classification since SVMs are used mostly in relevant literature.

During the test phase, the sensor signals were pre-processed and parameterized as during training. The SMO classification model was used to label each of the activities. In order to directly compare the proposed methodology with previous approaches evaluated on the same dataset, we followed the evaluation protocol applied in the existing literature [24–26, 38–40]. In particular, we used the existing random partitioning of the dataset into two sets, where 70% consists of training samples and 30% consists of test samples.

However, for the motion dependent classification scheme, in order to learn the weights for the fusion function (2), sensitivity values should be obtained based absolutely on the training set since an overlap with the test set would lead to over fitting. For this purpose, in order to obtain the appropriate weights for (2) we performed N times 10-fold cross validation on the N versions of the training set respectively.

5   Experimental Results

5.1   Evaluation of the Motion Dependent Classification Scheme

The motion dependent classification scheme presented in Sect. 3 was evaluated using the feature extraction and the classification algorithm described in Sect. 4. Initially, each motion dependent classification model $i (1 \leq i \leq N \, and \, N = 6)$ was evaluated on the corresponding version of the training set which treats the motion/ADL under consideration as positive class and all the others as negative. The aim of this evaluation is to obtain appropriate weights for the fusion function (2) which combines the individual decisions. For this purpose, the sensitivity of each model as defined in (1) was used. The obtained values for the sensitivity measure for each of the motion dependent classification models for the training set are tabulated in Table 3.

Table 3. Sensitivity of motion dependent classifiers on the training set.

Motion dependent classification model	Sensitivity
Walking-vs- all	100.00%
Walking-Upstairs-vs-all	99.53%
Walking-Downstairs-vs-all	99.49%
Sitting-vs-all	95.41%
Standing-vs-all	96.36%
Laying-vs-all	100.00%

Based on these values, the fusion function is:

$$Decision = 1d_1 + 1d_2 + 0.99d_4 + 0.95d_4 + 0.96d_5 + 1d_6. \qquad (3)$$

The classification performance of the overall framework was evaluated on the 30% of the dataset consisting of the testing samples in terms of accuracy defined as

$$Accuracy = \frac{TP + TN}{TP + FP + TN + FN}. \qquad (4)$$

where TP denotes the true positives, TN denotes the true negatives, FP the false positives and FN the false negatives. Table 4 shows the achieved accuracy obtained from the test set for the motion dependent binary classifiers and the proposed fusion framework. The achieved accuracy of the proposed scheme is 99%.

Table 4. Accuracy of motion dependent classifiers and fusion scheme on the test set.

Motion dependent classification model	Accuracy
Walking-vs- all	100.00%
Walking-Upstairs-vs-all	99.96%
Walking-Downstairs-vs-all	100.00%
Sitting-vs-all	99.10%
Standing-vs-all	99.15%
Laying-vs-all	100.00%
Proposed fusion framework	98.98%

5.2 Evaluation of the Multiclass Classification Scheme

In order to make a fair comparison of the proposed fusion scheme with the common multiclass classification scheme, we evaluated the latter after an attempt to optimize it either by feature selection or by performing subject dependent classification.

Feature Selection. Regarding the first optimization strategy, we applied feature ranking on the whole dataset (consisting of all available subjects) using the ReliefF algorithm as described in Sect. 3.2. The performance of the classification, in terms of accuracy, for different number of N-best features (N = 10, 20, 30, ..., 560) for the SMO algorithm is shown in Fig. 4.

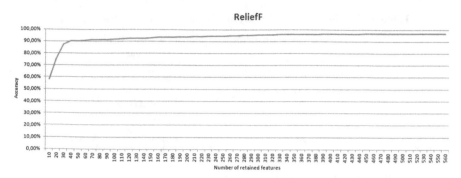

Fig. 4. Classification Accuracy for different subsets of N-best features (N = 10,20,..., 550) reproduced from [28].

As can be seen in Fig. 4 the highest classification accuracy is achieved when a large subset of discriminative features is used. Specifically, the highest accuracy is achieved for a subset of 550 best features with a percentage of 97% which is equal to the accuracy achieved when all features are used. It seems that the size and the variability of the dataset is relatively large requiring a feature vector of high dimensionality to accurately discriminate between the six classes. However, with only 40 features a high accuracy equal to 90% can be achieved.

Table 5 show the 40 best features according to the ReliefF ranking algorithm. Although it is best to use a high dimensional feature vector to achieve higher classification accuracy, feature selection still being important in cases where a light human motion identification module is needed such as in FRAILSAFE [27].

Table 5. ReliefF Feature Ranking reproduced from [28].

Ranking	Feauture
1	tGravityAcc_energy_X
2	fBodyAccJerk_entropy_X
3	fBodyAcc_entropy_X
4	fBodyAccJerk_entropy_Y
5	tBodyAccJerkMag_entropy
6	angle(X_gravityMean)
7	tGravityAcc_min_X
8	tGravityAcc_mean_X
9	tBodyAccJerk_entropy_X
10	tGravityAcc_max_X
11	fBodyBodyAccJerkMag_entropy
12	tBodyAcc_max_X
13	tBodyAccJerk_entropy_Y
14	fBodyAccMag_entropy

(continued)

Table 5. (*continued*)

Ranking	Feauture
15	fBodyAcc_entropy_Y
16	fBodyAccJerk_entropy_Z
17	tBodyAccJerk_entropy_Z
18	tBodyGyroJerkMag_entropy
17	tGravityAcc_energy_Y
20	tBodyAccMag_entropy
21	tGravityAccMag_entropy
22	tGravityAcc_mean_Y
23	tBodyGyroJerk_entropy_Z
24	tGravityAcc_max_Y
25	fBodyAcc_entropy_Z
26	tGravityAcc_entropy_Z
27	tGravityAcc_min_Y
28	fBodyGyro_entropy_X
29	fBodyGyro_entropy_X
30	tBodyGyroJerk_entropy_X
31	fBodyAcc_mad_X
32	fBodyAcc_std_X
33	tBodyAcc_std_Y
34	fBodyAcc_mad_Y
35	tBodyAcc_std_X
36	fBodyBodyGyroJerkMag_entropy
37	tBodyAcc_mad_Y
38	fBodyGyro_entropy_Y
39	tBodyGyroMag_entropy
40	fBodyAcc_std_Y

Subject Dependent Classification. Regarding the second optimization strategy, we trained subject specific classifiers as described in Sect. 3.2. The results are shown on Table 6.

As can be seen in Table 6, the overall highest accuracy of the proposed methodology for human motion identification is 100% for subjects 1, 9, 11,14, 23, 24, 26, 27 and 29 and the lowest accuracy 69.07% was obtained for the 6th subject. However, the mean accuracy is relatively high, i.e., 94.35%.

Comparison. Table 7 compares the proposed fusion scheme with the common multiclass classification scheme and other relevant approaches evaluated on the same dataset with the same evaluation protocol. As can be seen the proposed framework outperforms both the multiclass classification scheme and the previous approaches [24, 25, 38–40] reaching an accuracy of 99%. The improvement of the overall performance is owed to the fact that motion-specific SVM-based detectors were used, which are able to accurately model the specific characteristics of each motion type.

Table 6. Subject dependent human motion identification Accuracy reproduced from [28].

Subject	Accuracy
1	100.00%
2	98.89%
3	95.10%
4	98.95%
5	93.33%
6	69.07%
7	100.00%
8	71.43%
9	100.00%
10	95.45%
11	100.00%
12	75.00%
13	94.90%
14	100.00%
15	95.92%
16	97.25%
17	91.82%
18	90.83%
17	82.41%
20	94.34%
21	99.18%
22	97.92%
23	100.00%
24	100.00%
25	96.72%
26	100.00%
27	100.00%
28	96.49%
29	100.00%
30	95.61%

Table 7. Comparison of existing methods on the test set.

Relevant literature	Accuracy
Proposed fusion scheme	**98.98%**
Multiclass classification - Feature selection	97.00%
Multiclass classification - Subject dependent	94.35%
Anguita et al. [24, 25]	89.30%
Reiss et al. [37]	94.40%
Romera-Paredes et al. [38]	96.33%
Kastner et al. [39]	96.23%

Moreover, during model training, the SVM algorithm adapts it's kernel mapping parameters appropriately for each target motion type in order the corresponding feature vectors to be better discriminated by the ones of the other human body motion types.

6 Conclusions

We presented a methodology for human motion identification from multi-parametric sensor data acquired using accelerometers and gyroscopes, which will be used as part of an end-to-end system for sensing and predicting treatment of frailty and associated co-morbidities using advanced personalized models and advanced interventions. The methodology uses motion dependent binary classification models that classify separately the sensor signals and combine the individual decisions using a fusion function based on the sensitivity of each model to discriminate the examined class. The classification models were trained using feature vectors consisting of a large number of time and frequency domain features and SVMs to train and test the motion dependent classification models. The proposed scheme is compared against the common multi-class classification scheme after optimization of the latter through feature selection and subject dependent classification. All schemes were evaluated using multi-parametric data from 30 subjects. The proposed scheme reached an accuracy of approximately 99% which is higher than the one achieved by the multiclass classification scheme even after its optimization. Finally, the proposed scheme was compared against other relevant studies in the literature. The achieved accuracy is more than 2.5% higher than the ones reported in the previous approaches evaluated on the same dataset with the same evaluation protocol.

Acknowledgements. The research reported in the present paper was partially supported by the FrailSafe Project (H2020- PHC-21-2015-690140) "Sensing and predictive treatment of frailty and associated co-morbidities using advanced personalized models and advanced interventions", co-funded by the European Commission under the Horizon 2020 research and innovation program.

References

1. Morley, J.E., et al.: Frailty consensus: a call to action. J. Am. Med. Directors Assoc. **14**, 392–397 (2013)
2. Chen, X., Mao, G., Leng, S.X.: Frailty syndrome: an overview. Clin. Interv. Aging **9**, 433–441 (2014)
3. Abellan van Kan, G., et al.: The I.A.N.A Task Force on frailty assessment of older people in clinical practice. J. Nutr. Health Aging **12**, 29–37 (2008)
4. Mitnitski, A.B., Graham, J.E., Mogilner, A.J., Rockwood, K.: Frailty, fitness and late-life mortality in relation to chronological and biological age. BMC Geriatr. **2**, 1 (2002)
5. Morley, J.E., Haren, M.T., Rolland, Y., Kim, M.J.: Frailty. Med. Clin. North Am. **90**, 837–847 (2006)
6. Seacw Project. http://cordis.europa.eu/project/rcn/191786_en.html

7. Eldergames Project. http://cordis.europa.eu/project/rcn/80186_en.html
8. Kinoptim Project. http://cordis.europa.eu/project/rcn/106678_en.html
9. Mporas, I., Tsirka, V., Zacharaki, E.I., Koutroumanidis, M., Richardson, M., Megalooikonomou, V.: Seizure detection using EEG and ECG signals for computer-based monitoring, analysis and management of epileptic patients. Expert Syst. Appl. **42**, 3227–3233 (2015)
10. Doremi Project. http://cordis.europa.eu/project/rcn/110829_en.html
11. Alfred Project. http://cordis.europa.eu/project/rcn/110629_en.html
12. Home Sweet Home Project. http://cordis.europa.eu/project/rcn/191712_en.html
13. Mobiserv Project. http://cordis.europa.eu/project/rcn/93537_en.html
14. Fate Project. http://cordis.europa.eu/project/rcn/191694_en.html
15. Jia, Y.: Diatetic and exercise therapy against diabetes mellitus. In: 2nd International Conference on Intelligent Networks and Intelligent Systems, pp. 693–696 (2009)
16. Khan, A., Lee, Y., Lee, S.Y., Kim, T.: Triaxial accel-erometer-based physical-activity recognition via augmented-signal features and a hierarchical recognizer. IEEE Trans. Inf Technol. Biomed. **14**, 1166–1172 (2010)
17. Mantyjarvi, J., Himberg, J., Seppanen, T.: Recognizing human motion with multiple acceleration sensors. In: IEEE International Conference on Systems, Man and Cybernetics, vol. 2, pp. 747–752 (2001)
18. Sekine, M., Tamura, T., Akay, M., Fujimoto, T., Togawa, T., Fukui, Y.: Discrimination of walking patterns using wavelet-based fractal analysis. IEEE Trans. Neural Syst. Rehabil. Eng. **10**, 188–196 (2002)
19. Ermes, M., Parkka, J., Mantyjarvi, J., Korhonen, I.: Frequent bit pattern mining over tri-axial accelerometer data streams for recognizing human activities and detecting fall. Procedia Comput. Sci. **19**, 56–63 (2013)
20. Bernecker, T., Graf, F., Kriegel, H., Moennig, C.: Activity recognition on 3D accelerometer data. Technical Report (2012)
21. Karantonis, D.M., Narayanan, M.R., Mathie, M., Lovell, N.H., Celler, B.G.: Implementation of a real-time human movement classifier using a triaxial accelerometer for ambulatory monitoring. IEEE Trans. Inf Technol. Biomed. **10**, 156–167 (2006)
22. Zhang, M., Sawchuk, A.: A feature selection-based framework for human activity recognition using wearable multimodal sensors. In: Proceedings of the 6th International Conference on Body Area Networks, pp. 92–98 (2011)
23. Ravi, N., Dandekar, N., Mysore, P., Littman, M.L.: Activity recognition from accelerometer data. Am. Assoc. Artif. Intell. **5**, 1541–1546 (2005)
24. Anguita, D., Ghio, A., Oneto, L., Parra, X., Reyes-Ortiz, J.L.: A public domain dataset for human activity recognition using smartphones. In: 21th European Symposium on Artificial Neural Networks, Computational Intelligence and Machine Learning, pp. 437–442 (2013)
25. Anguita, D., Ghio, A., Oneto, L., Parra, X., Reyes-Ortiz, Jorge L.: Human activity recognition on smartphones using a multiclass hardware-friendly support vector machine. In: Bravo, J., Hervás, R., Rodríguez, M. (eds.) IWAAL 2012. LNCS, vol. 7657, pp. 216–223. Springer, Heidelberg (2012). doi:10.1007/978-3-642-35395-6_30
26. Reyes-Ortiz, J.L., Ghio, A., Parra, X., Anguita, D., Cabestany, J., Catala, A.: Human activity and motion disorder recognition: towards smarter interactive cognitive environments. In: 21th European Symposium on Artificial Neural Networks, Computational Intelligence and Machine Learning, pp. 403–412 (2013)
27. FrailSafe project: http://frailsafe-project.eu/

28. Pippa, E., Mporas, I., Megalooikonomou, V.: Feature selection evaluation for light human motion identification in frailty monitoring system. In: 2nd International Conference on Information and Communication Technologies for Ageing Well and e-Health (ICT4AWE) (2016)
29. Kononenko, I.: Estimating attributes: analysis and extension of RELIEF. Mach. Learn. **784**, 171–182 (2005)
30. Kira, K., Rendell, L.A.: A practical approach to feature selection. In: Proceedings of 9th International Conference on Machine Learning, pp. 249–256 (1992)
31. Dietterich, T.G.: Machine learning research: four current directions. Artif. Intell. Mag. **18**, 97–136 (1997)
32. Sun, Y., Wu, D.: A RELIEF based feature extraction algorithm. In: Proceedings of SIAM International Conference on Data Mining, pp. 188–195 (2008)
33. Sun, Y., Li, J.: Iterative RELIEF for feature weighting. In: Proceedings of 21st International Conference on Machine Learning, pp. 913–920 (2006)
34. Kononenko, I., Simec, E., Robnik-Sikonja, M.: Overcoming the myopic of inductive learning algorithms with RELIEF-F. Appl. Intell. **7**, 39–55 (1997)
35. Keerthi, S.S., Shevade, S.K., Bhattacharyya, C., Murthy, K.R.K.: Improvements to Platt's SMO algorithm for SVM classifier design. Neural Comput. **13**, 637–649 (2001)
36. Platt, J.: Fast training of support vector machines using sequential minimal optimization. Advances in Kernel Methods - Support Vector Learning, pp. 185–208 (1998)
37. Hall, M., Frank, E., Holmes, G., Pfahringer, B., Reutemann, P., Witten, I.H.: The WEKA data mining software: an update. SIGKDD Explor. **11**, 10–18 (2009)
38. Reiss, A., Hendeby, G., Stricker, D.: A competitive approach for human activity recognition on smartphones. In: European Symposium on Artificial Neural Networks. Computational Intelligence and Machine Learning, pp. 455–460 (2013)
39. Romera-Paredes, B., Aung, H., Bianchi-Berthouze, N.: A one-vs-one classifier ensemble with majority voting for activity recognition. In: European Symposium on Artificial Neural Networks, Computational Intelligence and Machine Learning, pp. 443–448 (2013)
40. Kastner, M., Strickert, M., Villmann, T.: A sparse kernelized matrix learning vector quantization model for human activity recognition. In: European Symposium on Artificial Neural Networks, Computational Intelligence and Machine Learning, pp. 449–454 (2013)

An Improved Scheme for Protecting Medical Data in Public Clouds

Nikos Fotiou and George Xylomenos$^{(\boxtimes)}$

Mobile Multimedia Laboratory, Department of Informatics,
School of Information Sciences and Technology,
Athens University of Economics and Business,
Patision 76, Athens 10434, Greece
{fotiou,xgeorge}@aueb.gr

Abstract. Public Clouds offer a convenient way for storing and sharing the large amounts of medical data that are generated by, for example, wearable health monitoring devices. Nevertheless, using a public infrastructure raises significant security and privacy concerns. Even if the data are stored in an encrypted form, the data owner should share some information with the Cloud provider in order to enable the latter to perform access control; given the high sensitivity of medical data, even such limited information may jeopardize end-user privacy. In this paper we employ an access control delegation scheme to enable the users themselves to perform access control on their data, even though these are stored in a public Cloud. In our scheme access control policies are evaluated by a user-controlled gateway and Cloud providers are only entrusted with respecting the gateway's decision. Furthermore, since medical data must often be shared with health providers of the user's choice, we rely on a proxy re-encryption technique to allow such sharing to take place. Our scheme encrypts data before storing them in the Cloud and applies proxy re-encryption using Cloud resources to encrypt data separately for each (authorized) user. Our proxy re-encryption scheme ensures that misbehaving Cloud providers cannot use re-encryption keys to share content with unauthorized clients, while delegating the costly re-encryption operations to the Cloud.

Keywords: Access control · Proxy re-encryption · Medical data · Public clouds

1 Introduction

Nowadays, smart devices that collect users' vital signals have become a commodity. It is expected that the data collected by these devices will soon be used for preventing and/or diagnosing various health related problems, as well as for promoting a healthier way of living and well-being. Storing and sharing these data using a public Cloud infrastructure appears to be an appealing option, as public Clouds offer cost effective, reliable and always-on storage services. On the

© Springer International Publishing AG 2017
C. Röcker et al. (Eds.): ICT4AWE 2016, CCIS 736, pp. 66–79, 2017.
DOI: 10.1007/978-3-319-62704-5_5

other hand, security and privacy concerns are raised, as medical data are highly sensitive and they should be very well protected, even against misbehavior by the Cloud service provider. Encryption and access control can be used as a countermeasure, but privacy threats remain. For example, an access control policy of the form "these (encrypted) data can only be accessed by psychiatrist A" reveals to the entity that performs access control that the data owner shares some data with a psychiatrist.

In this paper we propose a scheme that allows secure and private storage of medical records in the Cloud. Our scheme allows data owners to define access control policies and to enforce them by themselves. The Cloud provider is only responsible for storing data and for respecting the access control decisions of the data owner. Even if the Cloud provider misbehaves, the data remain protected, since they are encrypted so that only authorized users can access them; unauthorized users – including the Cloud provider – can learn nothing about the data. In order to achieve our goal we use the system proposed by [1] by adding an additional layer of data confidentiality protection.

Since our proposal encrypts data before storing them in the Cloud, they cannot be directly shared with authorized health providers, without revealing the user's encryption keys. To allow controlled data sharing, our scheme relies on re-encrypting the data before sharing, so that they can only be decrypted by users authorized by the data owner. Rather than having the user's devices re-encrypt data, we rely on a proxy re-encryption scheme so as to delegate this processing to the Cloud provider, without however allowing the Cloud provider to gain access to the encrypted data. In this manner, the user only needs to deal with the original data encryption, delegating all further storage and processing to the Cloud provider.

This paper extends our previously published work [2] in the following areas: (i) we improve our proxy re-encryption based scheme so as to protect our system against misbehaving Cloud providers, (ii) we add a client authentication procedure, (iii) we provide more details about our protocol, (iv) we perform a more thorough evaluation of our system, including its security evaluation.

The remainder of the paper is organized as follows. Section 2 briefly presents access control delegation and proxy re-encryption. Section 3 presents our system design in detail. In Sect. 4 we evaluate our solution and in Sect. 5 we present related work in the area. Finally, we conclude our paper in Sect. 6

2   Background

2.1   Access Control Delegation

The access control scheme proposed in [1] separates *data storage* and *access control* functions: the former is implemented in a public Cloud, whereas the latter is implemented by a trusted entity named the *access control provider* (ACP). These entities interact with each other as follows (Fig. 1)[1]: Initially, a data owner

---

[1] The description has been modified to fit the purposes of the present paper.

creates an *access control policy*, stores it in an ACP (step 1) and obtains a *URI* for that policy (step 2). Then, he stores some data in the Cloud, indicating at the same time the URI of the policy that protects these data (step 3). When a client tries to access these data (step 4), the Cloud responds with the URI of the access control policy and a unique token (step 5). Then, the client authenticates herself to the ACP and requests authorization (step 6). If the client "satisfies" the access control policy, the ACP generates a signed *authorization* and sends it back (step 7). Finally, the client repeats her request to the Cloud, this time including the authorization (step 8). The Cloud checks the validity of the authorization and if it is valid, it returns the desired data (step 9).

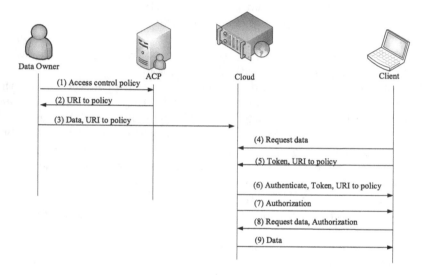

Fig. 1. Access control delegation (reproduced from [2]).

This scheme has many advantages. The Cloud provider learns nothing about the client since all her personal data (which are required to evaluate the access control policy) are stored in the ACP. Moreover, Cloud providers do not have to interpret any access control policies, therefore they do not need to understand content owner specific semantics. Each ACP can implement any conceivable access control policy, since the Cloud provider only sees the URI identifying the policy and the authorizations returned by the ACP. Access control policies are reusable i.e., in order to protect a new item using an existing access control policy the same URI can be simply re-used. Access control policies can be easily updated; updating and access control policy does not involve any communication with the Cloud provider. Finally, provided that many Cloud providers support this scheme, it is trivial for a data owner to migrate from one Cloud provider to another, as the URIs of the access control policies remain the same.

2.2   Proxy Re-encryption

A Proxy re-encryption (PRE) scheme is a scheme in which a third, semi-trusted party, the *proxy*, is allowed to alter a ciphertext encrypted with the public key of a user A (the delegator), in a way that another user B (the delegatee) can decrypt it with her own appropriate key (in most cases, her secret private key). During this process the proxy learns nothing about the private keys of A and B, and does not gain access to the encrypted data.

In this paper we employ the *identity-based proxy re-encryption* (IB-PRE) by Green and Ateniese [3]. In particular we use a variant of that scheme in which the delegatee uses public key based encryption (PKE) instead of identity-based encryption (Sect. 5 of [3]). This scheme specifies the following algorithms (the description has been adapted to the PKE variant):

- **Setup**: it is executed by a *Private Key Generator* (PKG). It takes as input a security parameter k and returns a **master-secret** key (MSK) and some **system parameters** (SP). The MSK is kept secret by the PKG, whereas the SP are made publicly available.
- **Extract**: it is executed by a PKG. It takes as input the SP, the MSK, and an identity ID, and returns a **secret** key SK_{ID}. An ID can be any arbitrary string.
- **Encrypt**: it can be executed by anyone. It takes as input an identity ID, a message M, and the SP, and returns a ciphertext C_{ID}. This ciphertext can only be decrypted by the owner of SK_{ID}, i.e., the secret key that corresponds to the identity ID.
- **RKGen**: it is executed by the owner of the identity $ID1$. It takes as input the SP, the secret key SK_{ID1} and the PKE public key PK_A of a user A. It outputs a re-encryption key $RK_{ID1 \to PK_A}$.
- **Reencrypt**: it is executed by a *proxy*. It takes as input the SP, a re-encryption key $RK_{ID1 \to PK_A}$, and a ciphertext C_{ID1} and outputs a new ciphertext C_{PK}, which can be decrypted by the owner of the PKE secret key SK_A.
- **Decrypt**: it is executed by the owner of the PKE secret key SK_A. It takes as input SP, C_{PK}, and SK_A, and returns the message M.

Figure 2 gives an example of a complete IB-PRE transaction. In this figure, initially the PKG generates the MSK and the SP, and makes the SP publicly available, while keeping the MSK to itself (step 1). This initializes the system. When a user $ID1$ wants to use the system, it asks the PKG to thect the secret key SK_{ID1} and return it to user $ID1$ (step 2). Another user $ID3$ can then encrypt a piece of text using the publicly known identity of $ID1$, creating a ciphertext C_{ID1}, which is then stored in a proxy (step 3). This ciphertext can only be decrypted by the user that owns $ID1$, and therefore knows the corresponding SK_{ID1}. To allow another user $ID2$ to decrypt the content using a PKE private key SK_{RSA_2}, the owner of $ID1$ creates a re-encryption key $RK_{ID1 \to RSA2}$ using the well known PKE public key PK_{RSA_2} of user $ID2$ and sends it to the proxy (step 4). The proxy re-encrypts C_{ID1} using the re-encryption key and generates C_{ID2} (step 5). The owner of SK_{RSA_2} is now able to decrypt the re-encrypted

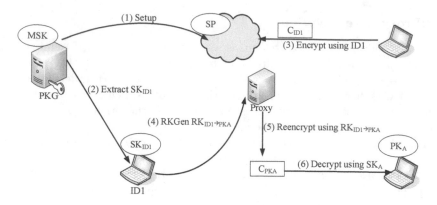

Fig. 2. IB-PRE example (adapted from [2]).

ciphertext (step 6). The proxy learns nothing about the contents of the ciphertext or the secret keys of the users.

If the original version of the scheme is used (instead of the PKE variant described above) then the secret keys of delegatees should be generated by a PKG. This however raises security concerns, since the PKG will know the private keys of all users. Although this is not a problem in some scenarios, in our case a delegatee is a doctor or a hospital that has access to very sensitive information. Therefore, this is an unacceptable security threat. Moreover, if a delegatee interacts with many delegators (as, for example, in the case of a hospital that interacts with its patients) then this results in a non-negligible key management overhead. For this reason, we rely instead on the PKE keys of the delegatees for the re-encryption procedures.

3   Design

In this section, we explain how the aforementioned access control and proxy re-encryption schemes are adapted for our scheme. We assume the use of smart devices that collect user related data, such as smart watches that measure cardio activity. All collected data are stored in a public Cloud. The smart devices do not interact directly with the Cloud; they instead communicate with a user controlled *gateway*. This gateway holds the roles of both the PKG and the ACP described in the previous section, i.e., the gateway generates the appropriate secret keys and is responsible for enforcing access control policies. In addition, a gateway is responsible for initially encrypting (not re-encrypting) files, storing them in the Cloud, and for generating re-encryption keys. Clients interested in receiving a file stored in the Cloud, initially send an unauthorized request to the Cloud provider. The Cloud provider re-directs them to the appropriate gateway, where they authenticate themselves and get authorized to access the protected file. The authorization process also results in the creation of an appropriate re-encryption key, which is securely transmitted to the Cloud provider. Then, clients issue authorized requests and receive the (re-encrypted) file. All communications (between the smart devices and the gateway, between the gateway and the Cloud, between the clients and the Cloud, and between the clients and the gateway) are secured using TLS. Figure 3 gives an overview of our system entities and their interactions, which we explain in more detail in the following subsections.

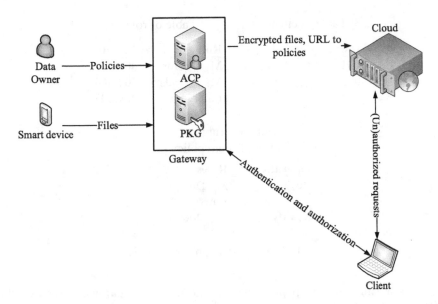

Fig. 3. An overview of the entities of our scheme and their interactions (adapted from [2]).

3.1 Setup

With this procedure a data owner creates access control policies and generates the appropriate cryptographic keys. Our system uses NIST's core Role-based Access Control (core-RBAC) model [4]. Based on this model, data owners create tables of clients, roles, and permissions. The table of clients contains tuples of the form $[index, identity]$ where $index$ is an integer number unique for each client and $identity$ is the client's public key. The table of roles contains tuples of the form $[role, <client_{index}>]$, where $role$ is a unique role name, and $<client_{index}>$ is a list of indices from the clients table and represents the clients that hold that specific role. Finally, for each file, the client maintains a table of permissions that contain tuples of the form $[operation, <role>]$, where $operation$ is an operation over the file (e.g., read, write, delete) and $<role>$ is a list of roles that are permitted to perform that operation. Each permission table is identified by a unique URI_{policy}. All relationships in a core-RBAC model are many-to-many, hence, a client may have multiple roles and a role may be allowed to perform multiple operations.

Figure 4 illustrates an example of access control policy definition. In this example, a data owner has defined three clients and three roles. It can be observed that client 003 has multiple roles. The data owner has created a permissions table and has specified its URI_{policy}. We can observe in this table that the role "My Doctors" is allowed to perform multiple operations.

Table of clients

Index	Identity
001	PK_{001}
002	PK_{002}
003	PK_{003}

Table of roles

Role	Clients
My Doctors	001
My Friends	002,003
Emergency	001,003

Permission Table
https://gw.example.com/policy32B

Operation	Roles
Read	My Doctors, Emergency
Modify	My Doctors

Fig. 4. Access control policy example.

The first time the setup procedure is executed, the gateway executes the IB-PRE `setup` algorithms and generates a master secret key (MSK) and the corresponding (public) system parameters. The MSK is securely stored in the gateway.

3.2   Data Storage

Data storage in the Cloud is achieved using the following steps:

– For each file that arrives in the gateway a permissions table and an appropriate URI_{policy} is generated, or an existing one may be re-used.
– The gateway generates a symmetric encryption key K, encrypts the file using K (we refer to the output of this encryption as $Enc_K(file)$), and encrypts K using the IB-PRE *encrypt* algorithm, using URI_{policy} as the input identity (we refer to the output of this encryption as $C_{URI_{policy}}(K)$).
– The gateway stores $Enc_K(file)$, $C_{URI_{policy}}(K)$, and URI_{policy} in the Cloud.

Gateways keep track of all files and their associated URI_{policy} and Cloud provider in a *table of files*. A table of files contains a set of tuples of the form $[filename, policy, Pub_{CP}]$ where $filename$ is the file name, $policy$ is the URI_{policy} of the file's permissions table, and Pub_{CP} is the public key of the Cloud provider where the file is stored. Cloud providers maintain a similar table that contains entries of the form $[filename, policy, Pub_{GW}]$, where Pub_{GW} is the public key of the gateway.

3.3   Unauthorized Request

This procedure is executed by a client in order to perform an operation over some protected data. The client sends an operation request to the Cloud provider that contains nothing but the operation itself and the name of the file it concerns. Upon receiving the request the Cloud provider creates a unique *token* (i.e., an adequately large random number) and sends it back to the client, along with the corresponding URI_{policy}. Cloud providers keep track of all generated tokens, as well as their associated URI_{policy}.

3.4   Client Authentication and Authorization

This procedure is executed by a client upon receiving a response to an unauthorized request. The client generates an authorization request that is composed of the following fields: URI_{policy}, *token*, *filename* (i.e., the name of the desired file), *operation*, Pub_{CP}, Pub_{Client} (i.e., the public key of the client), and digitally sings this message using his private key (we refer to the outcome of the signature operation as $Sign_{Client}(msg)$). Then, the client sends the authorization request to the gateway denoted by URI_{policy}. Upon receiving this request, the gateway performs the following steps in order to authorize the client:

- It verifies $Sign_{Client}(msg)$. If the signature verification fails, the client is not authorized, as he has not proved his identity.
- From the files table it retrieves the *policy* and the Pub_{CP} of the entry that corresponds to the *filename* included in the authorization request and checks if these fields match those included in the request. If this verification fails, the client is not authorized.
- It retrieves the file's permissions table and examines if the client identified by Pub_{Client} has a role authorized to perform the operation included in the authorization request. If this verification fails, the client is not authorized.

If the client is authorized, then the gateway performs the following operations:

- It executes the IB-PRE RKGen algorithm and creates $RK_{URI_{policy} \rightarrow Pub_{client}}$ and encrypts this key using Pub_{CP}. We refer to the output of the latter encryption as $C_{CP}(RK)$.
- It sends to the client an authorization response which contains $C_{CP}(RK)$ and a digital signature generated using the gateway's private key that covers $C_{CP}(RK)$ and all fields of the authorization request, except Pub_{Client} and $Sign_{Client}(msg)$. We refer to that signature as $Sign_{GW}(msg)$.

3.5   Authorized Request

This procedure is executed by an authorized client. The client constructs an authorized request that includes the following fields: the *filename* of the desired file, the *operation*, the *token* received with the execution of the *unauthorized request* procedure, and the authorization response retrieved with the execution of the *client authentication and authorization* procedure. Then, the client sends this request to the Cloud provider. Upon receiving this request, the Cloud provider performs the following steps in order to decide if the client is permitted to perform the requested operation:

- It retrieves URI_{policy} and Pub_{GW} that corresponds to the *name* and examines if the retrieved URI_{policy} matches the one associated with the token. If it does not match, the client is authorized.
- It evaluates $Sign_{GW}(msg)$. If the signature verification fails, the client is not authorized.

If the client is permitted to perform the requested operation, the Cloud provider performs the following operations:

- It uses $RK_{URI_{policy}\rightarrow Pub_{client}}$ and the IB-PRE `Reencrypt` algorithm to re-encrypt $C_{URI_{policy}}(K)$ so as to generate $C_{Client}(K)$.
- It sends $C_{Client}(K)$ and $Enc_K(file)$ back to the client.

Figure 5 illustrates a message sequence diagram of the unauthorized request, client authentication and authorization, and authorized request procedures.

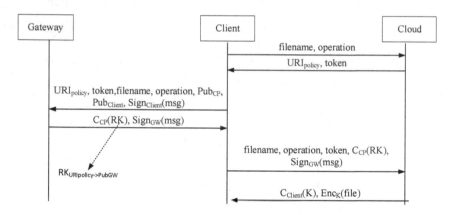

Fig. 5. Message sequence diagram.

3.6 External Roles

When protecting medical data stored in the Cloud, it is desirable to have roles, and create access control policies based on such roles, which are defined by external (third) parties. For example, "doctors of hospital A" could be such a role, defined by the entity "hospital A". Contemporary cryptographic techniques such as attributed-based encryption [5], or hierarchical identity-based encryption [6] could be used to achieve this goal. However, we do not consider this option, because, for security reasons, we want each client to be able to generate her keys by herself, which is not possible with these cryptographic techniques. Moreover, these cryptographic techniques have been found to be ineffective when used for controlling access to data stored in the Cloud [7]. Instead, we follow a more conservative approach. We assume that each role is identified by a public key, generated by the same third party that has defined this role. This key is used by data owners in the table of roles instead of $< client_{index} >$. Moreover, the public key of each client is included in a X.509 certificate which is digitally signed using the private key of the role. For instance, in our example the public keys of the doctors should be signed by the private key of the role "doctors of hospital A". If a client has multiple roles, he should have multiple X.509 certificates.

When a client requests authorization from the gateway, she includes in her request her digital certificate. The digital signature included in the certificate is used by the gateway in order to evaluate whether or not the client belongs to an authorized role. If this is the case, then the gateway can use the public key of the client (included in the certificate) to generate the appropriate re-encryption key (as described in the previous section), and therefore to allow her to access the protected file. Note that the gateway does not need to know or store any details about the members of an external role; it only needs to know the public key of that role. In our example, this allows a hospital to change the set of doctors that it has authorized, without communicating with all the gateways of the clients that trust the hospital.

4   Evaluation

We have implemented the IB-PRE part of our system by modifying the Green-Atenicse IB-PRE implementation included in the Charm Crypto library [8] to support PKE for the delegatee. In particular, we have added support for the Cramer and Shoup elliptic curve based public key cryptosystem [9]. That is, in our implementation a ciphertext generated using Identity-based encryption is transformed into a ciphertext that can be decrypted using a Cramer-Shoup secret key (combined with some pairing operations).

In order to achieve a security level equivalent to RSA with a key size of 1024 bits for the encryption of the symmetric key, the size of SP is 2048 bits, the size of $C_{URI_{policy}}(K)$ is 2048 bits, and the size of a re-encryption key is 2816 bits. In Table 1 we report the time required to perform various cryptographic operations, in an Xbuntu 14.04 Desktop machine, running in a single core of an Intel i5-4440 3.1 GHz processor with 2GB of RAM, using the Charm Crypto library v0.43, python v2.7, the pbc library v0.5.4, and the gmp library v5.1.3.

The IB-PRE cryptographic algorithm used by our system has been proven to be secure in [3]. Each data item is encrypted using a different symmetric encryption key, therefore the compromise of a symmetric encryption key would require the re-encryption of only that specific item with a fresh key. This is an inevitable overhead of all similar systems and it is due to the fact that public key encryption cannot be applied directly to the file contents, due to its computational complexity. Nevertheless, for small data items, such as readings from wearable devices, it may be possible to negate the need for symmetric encryption.

Table 1. Computation overhead of IB-PRE cryptographic operations.

Operation	time in ms
Create $C_{URI_{policy}}(K)$	23
Generate $RK_{URI_{policy} \to Pub_{client}}$	40
Re-encrypt $C_{URI_{policy}}(K)$	4
Decrypt $C_{Client}(K)$	25

Traditional proxy re-encryption schemes require proxies to be semi-trusted, i.e., a proxy should (i) not share re-encryption keys, and (ii) use re-encryption keys only for authorized users. Our system relaxes the second requirement: since symmetric encryption keys are encrypted using URI_{policy} as an input identity a $RK_{URI_{policy} \to Pub_{client}}$ would be useful for clients that abide by URI_{policy}. In other words, if a client does not abide by an access control policy, the gateway will never generate the corresponding re-encryption key.

Client revocation is achieved by removing a client from a role, or by removing a role from a permission. From the moment a client is disallowed to perform an operation, a gateway will not generate a re-encryption key when that client requests authorization for this operation. Nevertheless, if the Cloud provider caches re-encryption keys and it is not trusted to use them properly, then the URI_{policy} of the permission table from which the client has been removed, has to be updated. As a consequence, a new $C_{URI_{policy}}(K)$ will have to be generated.

Our system borrows most of the properties of the access control delegation scheme described in [1]. In particular, our system is generic enough, it can be easily implemented by a Cloud provider, data can be easily transferred between Cloud providers that implement this solution, it protects client privacy against Cloud providers, and it allows easy modification of access control policies. Compared to [1], our system does not hide the Client's interests from the ACP. This happens because we use URI_{policy} for protecting content confidentiality, hence it is not possible to use different a URI_{policy} for each operation (as in [1]). If hiding the Client's interests is highly desirable, then the "level extension" (Sect. 3.5 in [1]) can be used.

Another notable difference of the present system compared to [1] is that the present system does not rely on an external mechanism for authenticating clients to ACPs, using instead a digital signature (i.e., $Sign_{Client}(msg)$). In order to prevent malicious users from re-using an authentication message, ACPs should keep track of already seen tokens. Nevertheless, even if this not possible, or this check fails, the malicious user will end up receiving a file that he cannot access.

5   Related Work

Löhr et al. [10] have proposed a solution for securing e-health clouds based on *Trusted Virtual Domains* (TVDs). TVD is a virtualization technique that creates secure "sandboxes" where user data can reside. This solution is orthogonal to our system: the solution by Löhr et al. concerns the design of secure clouds specific to e-health services, whereas our solution assumes a generic cloud service and builds a secure data sharing system on top of it.

Wu et al. [11] propose an access control mechanism for sharing electronic health records in the Cloud. The main component of their mechanism is an *access broker* that is responsible for enforcing access control policies. The access broker is an entity shared among many stakeholders, therefore, privacy concerns are raised. In our work, access control policies are enforced by data owners in a way that reveals no information about data owners or clients to third parties (including the Cloud provider). Son et al. [12] propose a mechanism that supports "dynamic" access control, i.e., access control that takes into consideration the user's context. In their solution, access control is also implemented in the Cloud, therefore the same privacy concerns are raised.

Fabian et al. [13] use attribute-based encryption (ABE) to protect medical data stored in multi-Cloud environments and shared among different cooperative organizations. ABE produces encrypted data in a way that only users with specific "attributes" can decrypt. In essence, ABE incorporates access control policies into ciphertexts. The disadvantage of using ABE for this purpose is that the loss of a private key that corresponds to an attribute requires the generation of a new key, the distribution of this key to all users that have this attribute, and the appropriate encryption of all files protected by this attribute. In contrast, in our system the loss of the data owner's secret key only requires a new encryption of all symmetric keys. Similarly, [14–16] use attribute-based encryption to protect personal health records stored in public cloud environments; these solution also suffer from the same problems.

Thilakanathan et al. [17] use ElGamal public key encryption and a proxy re-encryption like protocol to protect generic health data stored in the cloud. Their solution relies on a centralized trusted third party that generates private keys on behalf of users. In our system users generate their private keys by themselves, therefore our approach offers increased security.

6   Conclusion and Future Work

In this paper we presented a scheme that allows secure and privacy preserving storage of medical data in public Clouds. Our solution combines access control delegation and proxy re-encryption, providing content confidentiality, client privacy enhancement, and resilience against malicious entities. This is achieved by following a gateway-based design, where a user-controlled gateway is responsible for encrypting user generated data, authenticating clients and enforcing access control policies. Cloud providers learn no information about the identity of the clients accessing the protected data and they are only trusted have to respect the gateway's decisions. Moreover, our proxy re-encryption based confidentiality solution protects sensitive data against misbehaving Cloud providers, even those that do not respect the gateway's access control decisions. Our proof of concept implementation shows that our solution is feasible, posing minimal overhead.

Future work involves the transfer of the encryption process to the devices that generate the data. In this manner, the device could store the data directly to the Cloud, avoiding the gateway, therefore reducing communication overhead. In this setup, the gateway would still hold the ACP and PKG roles. Moreover, the ACP could also be used for authenticating end-user devices to the Cloud.

References

1. Fotiou, N., Machas, A., Polyzos, G.C., Xylomenos, G.: Access control as a service for the cloud. J. Internet Serv. Appl. **6**, 1–15 (2015)
2. Fotiou, N., Xylomenos, G.: Protecting medical data stored in public clouds. In: Proceedings of the 2nd International Conference on Information and Communication Technologies for Ageing Well and e-Health (ICT4AWE) (2016)
3. Green, M., Ateniese, G.: Identity-based proxy re-encryption. In: Katz, J., Yung, M. (eds.) ACNS 2007. LNCS, vol. 4521, pp. 288–306. Springer, Heidelberg (2007). doi:10.1007/978-3-540-72738-5_19
4. Ferraiolo, D.F., Sandhu, R., Gavrila, S., Kuhn, D.R., Chandramouli, R.: Proposed nist standard for role-based access control. ACM Trans. Inf. Syst. Secur. **4**, 224–274 (2001)
5. Goyal, V., Pandey, O., Sahai, A., Waters, B.: Attribute-based encryption for fine-grained access control of encrypted data. In: Proceedings of the 13th ACM Conference on Computer and Communications Security, pp. 89–98 (2006)
6. Boneh, D., Boyen, X., Goh, E.-J.: Hierarchical identity based encryption with constant size ciphertext. In: Cramer, R. (ed.) EUROCRYPT 2005. LNCS, vol. 3494, pp. 440–456. Springer, Heidelberg (2005). doi:10.1007/11426639_26
7. Garrison III., W.C., Shull, A., Myers, S., Lee, A.J.: On the practicality of cryptographically enforcing dynamic access control policies in the cloud. In: Proceedings of the IEEE Symposium on Security and Privacy (2016)
8. Akinyele, J., Garman, C., Miers, I., Pagano, M., Rushanan, M., Green, M., Rubin, A.: Charm: a framework for rapidly prototyping cryptosystems. J. Cryptogr. Eng. **3**, 111–128 (2013)
9. Cramer, R., Shoup, V.: A practical public key cryptosystem provably secure against adaptive chosen ciphertext attack. In: Krawczyk, H. (ed.) CRYPTO 1998. LNCS, vol. 1462, pp. 13–25. Springer, Heidelberg (1998). doi:10.1007/BFb0055717
10. Löhr, H., Sadeghi, A.R., Winandy, M.: Securing the e-health cloud. In: Proceedings of the 1st ACM International Health Informatics Symposium, pp. 220–229 (2010)
11. Wu, R., Ahn, G.J., Hu, H.: Secure sharing of electronic health records in clouds. In: Proceedings of the 8th International Conference on Collaborative Computing: Networking, Applications and Worksharing (CollaborateCom), pp. 711–718 (2012)
12. Son, J., Kim, J.D., Na, H.S., Baik, D.K.: Dynamic access control model for privacy preserving personalized healthcare in cloud environment. Technol. Health Care **24**, 123–129 (2015)
13. Fabian, B., Ermakova, T., Junghanns, P.: Collaborative and secure sharing of healthcare data in multi-clouds. Inf. Syst. **48**, 132–150 (2015)
14. Akinyele, J.A., Pagano, M.W., Green, M.D., Lehmann, C.U., Peterson, Z.N., Rubin, A.D.: Securing electronic medical records using attribute-based encryption on mobile devices. In: Proceedings of the 1st ACM Workshop on Security and Privacy in Smartphones and Mobile Devices, pp. 75–86 (2011)

15. Li, M., Yu, S., Zheng, Y., Ren, K., Lou, W.: Scalable and secure sharing of personal health records in cloud computing using attribute-based encryption. IEEE Trans. Parallel Distrib. Syst. **24**, 131–143 (2013)
16. Liu, J., Huang, X., Liu, J.K.: Secure sharing of personal health records in cloud computing: ciphertext-policy attribute-based signcryption. Future Gener. Comput. Syst. **52**, 67–76 (2015)
17. Thilakanathan, D., Chen, S., Nepal, S., Calvo, R., Alem, L.: A platform for secure monitoring and sharing of generic health data in the cloud. Future Gener. Comput. Syst. **35**, 102–113 (2014)

A Technological Framework for EHR Interoperability: Experiences from Italy

Mario Ciampi[1]([✉]), Mario Sicuranza[1], Angelo Esposito[1,2], Roberto Guarasci[3,4], and Giuseppe De Pietro[1]

[1] Institute for High Performance Computing and Networking, National Research Council of Italy, Naples, Italy
{mario.ciampi,mario.sicuranza,angelo.esposito,
giuseppe.depietro}@na.icar.cnr.it
[2] Department of Engineering, University of Naples Parthenope, Naples, Italy
[3] Institute for Informatics and Telematics, National Research Council of Italy, Rende, CS, Italy
[4] Department of Linguistics, University of Calabria, Rende, CS, Italy
roberto.guarasci@unical.it

Abstract. Electronic Health Records (EHRs) systems enable the construction of longitudinal collection of health information about individual patients, by integrating health data produced by the healthcare facilities. The advantags associated with the use of such systems are in terms of improvement of quality of care and cost reduction. An important barrier to the availability of exhaustive longitudinal collections of health data is represented by the lack of interoperability among EHR systems. In Italy, each region has been developing its own EHR systems according to the national guidelines and technical specifications compliant to the indications provided by a Italian Law issued in 2012 and updated in 2013. This paper describes the national technological framework designed from a National Technical Board for making interoperable the regional EHR systems each other, preserving the privacy of the patients. The framework, based on a System-of-Systems approach, enables healthcare professionals both to (i) consult health documents associated with a patient, even if they are produced in other regions, and (ii) register new health documents for patients assisted by other regions.

Keywords: Electronic health record · Interoperability · Framework · Italy

1   Introduction

The use of ICT in healthcare has resulted in a considerable development of health information systems (HISs) in order to both enhance the quality of care services, and simultaneously reduce costs [15,25]; the most important example of HIS is the Electronic Health Record (EHR), which allows a fast exchange of clinical data between different healthcare organizations. In the last decades, many

C. Röcker et al. (Eds.): ICT4AWE 2016, CCIS 736, pp. 80–99, 2017.
DOI: 10.1007/978-3-319-62704-5_6

countries in the world have made significant efforts to develop EHR systems [13]. The International Organization for Standardization (ISO) defines EHR as a repository of patient data in digital form, stored and exchanged securely, and accessible by multiple authorized users. It contains retrospective, concurrent and prospective information and its primary purpose is to support continuing, efficient and quality integrated health care.

Despite such efforts in the realization of EHRs, the systems developed, at different levels (for example regional and national), are very often not able to interoperate each other [24], due to a plethora of reasons. First, each country or regional domain is characterized by its own legal requirements, especially about privacy protection. Second, countries or regions have typically different needs, depending on their dimension, number of citizens, number of healthcare facilities, etc. Finally, the development of the systems have been started in different periods, adopting or applying diverse standards in different ways [20].

The lack of interoperability among these systems can result in decreased levels of quality of patient care and waste of financial resources. In fact, when a patient benefits from a health service outside her/his health care domain, the health professional that treats the patient is not able to access the patient health information, due to the impossibility of cooperation between the EHR system used by the health professional and the one related to the patient. Therefore, the health professional typically requires the patient to repeat a clinical exam already executed. With respect to interoperability, several levels of interoperability are defined in literature [22]: *technical interoperability*, for which the systems share the communication protocols making possible, e.g., the exchange of bytes between them; *syntactic interoperability*, which aims at making the systems capable of communicating and exchanging data through the sharing of data formats; *semantic interoperability*, whose purpose is to enable systems to exchange data and interpret the information exchanged in the same way; *organizations & services interoperability*, where business processes are shared between the systems.

The importance of making EHR systems able to interoperate each other has motivated by the increase of the phenomenon of the patient mobility for reasons of care. For example, we can consider Italy where 570k hospitalizations are made by patients in a region different from that they reside only in 2015 [1]. In Italy, the autonomy about healthcare delivered by the Italian Constitution to each region caused the spread of heterogeneous regional EHR systems. After some national initiatives aimed at proposing a first architectural model at national level, the emanation of Italian norms has allowed defining both (i) the national architectural model of reference, and (ii) the functional and privacy requirements to be respected by all the Italian regions.

This paper, extending the concepts illustrated in a previous work [18], describes the Italian architecture for EHR system interoperability, developed by a National Technical Board, coordinated by the Agency for Digital Italy (AgID) and the Ministry of Health, with the technical support of the National Research Council of Italy (CNR) and the participation of the Ministry of Economy and Finance and Italian regions.

This paper is organized as follows. Section 2 provides some background and related work on the main standards, projects on e-health data interoperability and the description of the Italian context. Section 3 describes the main features of the national infrastructure for EHR systems, highlighting the cross-border business processes. Section 4 provides some technical details about the architecture of EHR systems and security issues. Finally, Sect. 5 concludes the paper with some final remarks and indications for future works.

2 Background and Related Work

2.1 Health Informatics Interoperability Standards

In order to achieve interoperability, the use of standards is a mandatory requirement. This section briefly describes the main health informatics standards, such HL7 and CEN ISO EN13606, and several initiatives, such openEHR and IHE, that promote the use of standards for health information systems development and integration.

The CEN/ISO EN13606 is a European norm from the European Committee for Standardization (CEN) also approved as an international ISO standard. It is designed to achieve semantic interoperability in the electronic health record communication. The overall goal of the CEN ISO 13606 standard is to define a rigorous and stable information architecture for communicating part or all of an electronic health record among EHR systems, or between EHR systems and a centralized EHR data repository [2].

Health Level Seven International (HL7) [3] is a non-profit organization involved in the development of international health informatics interoperability standards. The goal of these standards is supporting the exchange, integration, sharing and retrieval of electronic health information. HL7 messaging standards define the language and data structure required for information integration among HISs. Version 2 of the standard (HL7 v2) is currently implemented in numerous health organizations, whereas Version 3 (HL7 v3) is based on an object-oriented model called *Reference Information Model* (RIM). Clinical Document Architecture (CDA) is a standard derived from the RIM with the aim of specifying clinical documents structure and semantics. Currently, HL7 is involved in the definition of a new health interoperability standard, named Fast Healthcare Interoperability Resources (FHIR), which combines the best features of the previous versions [4].

openEHR [5] is an international not-for-profit foundation, which issued a detailed and tested specification for an interoperable HIS platform. Such a vision of openEHR had a significant influence on the development of the healthcare industry standards, such as HL7 and CEN EN1360610, with recommendations for an interoperable interconnection of HISs. OpenEHR consists of a generic information reference model, application-specific archetypes [14] and context-specific templates.

Integrate the Healthcare Enterprise (IHE) is an international initiative founded by Radiological Society of North America (RSNA) and Healthcare Information and Management Systems Society (HIMSS) with the goal of supporting the integration of HISs through existing standards. IHE promotes the coordinated use of established standards such as HL7 to address specific clinical needs in support of optimal patient care. IHE constantly defines Integration Profiles within Technical Frameworks, to provide definitions on the implementation of health standards in order to meet clinical needs and solve problems related to specific use cases: a known example of a Technical Framework is the *IHE IT Infrastructure Technical Framework*. In this context, the integration profile more relevant in the IT Infrastructure domain is Cross-Enterprise Document Sharing (XDS), which has the scope of facilitating the sharing of patient electronic health records across health enterprises [6]. IHE XDS aims at facilitating the sharing of clinical documents within an affinity domain (a group of healthcare facilities that intend to work together) by storing documents in an ebXML registry/repository architecture.

2.2 Health Interoperability Projects

This subsection describes the most relevant international interoperability projects on the development of EHR systems.

Canada Health Infoway is an independent, federally-funded, not-for-profit organization with the responsibility of accelerating the adoption of digital health solutions across Canada. Along with the Canadian provinces and territories, Infoway provided a national framework called EHR blackprint, with the aim of guiding the development of the systems in each different province. The key elements of the framework, built following a Service-Oriented Architecture (SOA) based on the HL7 Version 3 standard, are: gateways, data repositories, registry services, infostructure, access mechanisms [7].

U.S. Healtheway (now Sequoia) is a non profit, public-private partnership that operationally supports the eHealth Exchange project. With production starting in 2007, eHealth Exchange has become a rapidly growing community of public and private organizations, with the aim of facilitating the exchange of health information in a trusted, secure, and scalable manner. The exchange is realized through Web Services conforming to specifications based on IHE integration profiles. Finally, in order to support the health information exchange at local and national level, an open-source software named CONNECT has been developed [8].

epSOS project was an European project aimed at promoting the interoperability among the EHR systems of EU Member States. The scope of the epSOS project, which involved 25 different European countries, was to realize a large-scale pilot testing the cross-border sharing of two kinds of health documents: patient summary and electronic prescription. To achieve such an objective, a service infrastructure was designed, built, and evaluated. The national EHR systems communicate each other by means of gateways, named National Contact Points (NCPs), by exchanging: (i) messages based on IHE specifications, and (ii) clinical documents in the HL7 CDA format [9]. Starting from the results achieved in the epSOS project, the projects *Simple European Networked Electronic Services (e-SENS)* and *Expanding Health Data Interoperability Services (EXPAND)* have been activated. The e-SENS project covers different aspects of ICT applied to cross-border processes in domains such as e-Health, e-Justice, e-Procurement and business setup; it goes towards the idea of the European Digital Market. The EXPAND project is characterized by a network of 16 EU Member States with the aim of moving towards an environment of sustainable cross-border European services, through the Connecting Europe Facility (CEF) at European level and the development of national infrastructures and services.

2.3   Italian Context

This subsection describes the Italian context about eHealth. The Italian Government, since 2003, has identified a number of general objectives for the national health service in the light of changes in the social panorama and the national policy, with the basic requirement to guarantee citizens health protection, social security, and equity, quality and transparency in the care. These national plans have enabled various regional systems to develop independently infrastructure and services for e-health. In fact, in Italy there are different regions (provinces and autonomous), each of which with its health autonomy.

The Italian regions, driven by different needs, have developed services for e-health independently. In this way, highly heterogeneous and hardly interoperable systems have been obtained. The "e-Government Plan 2012" made by the Italian Ministry for Public Administration and Innovation has defined a set of digital innovation projects to modernize and make more efficient and transparent public administration, in order to promote the simplification and digitization of primary health care services.

A reference model was developed in the "Electronic Health Records guidelines" approved by a National Technical Board. The guidelines produced are compliant to the national normative and to the European strategic approach, according to which the role of the citizen-patient has a central value [21]. In Italy, a first prototypal architectural model for the realization of an interoperability secure EHR infrastructure, named InFSE [19], was defined and developed within three conjunct projects between the Department of Technological Innovation of the Presidency of the Council of Ministers and CNR.

The infrastructure, in absence of a norm, was designed with the aim of enabling interoperability among regional EHR systems. The components of the infrastructure were implemented and used in experimentations that have had the scope of enable the interchange of clinical documents by means of the interoperability of some regional EHR systems. The software components of the InFSE infrastructure were also used within the national IPSE project linked to epSOS, in which 10 Italian regions were involved. The aim of the project was to make regional EHR systems able to interoperate each other for the interchange of patient summaries.

The Laws 179/2012 and 98/2013, and the subsequent decree DPCM 178/2015 (Decree 178, 2015), have provided the Italian legal system of a definition of EHR, meant as the set of digital health and social-health data and documents generated from present and past clinical events, about the patient. According to the norms, EHR can be used for three finalities: (a) prevention, diagnosis, treatment and rehabilitation; (b) study and scientific research in the medical, biomedical and epidemiological field; (c) health planning, verification of the quality of care and evaluation of health care. The decree DPCM of 29 September 2015 n. 178 defines the rules by which the Italian regions have to set up their EHR systems.

The regulatory framework has permitted to a National Technical Board to define a set of reference guidelines for the implementation of the EHR systems [17]. Then, a set of technical specifications, which establish the main requirements to be met by the regions, have been defined to guarantee interoperability at different levels:

- *technical interoperability* is assured by sharing communication protocols among services interfaces;
- *syntactic interoperability* is reached by the use of common data formats;
- *semantic interoperability* is guaranteed by adopting both same data formats and coding systems;
- *organizations & services interoperability* is enabled by the sharing of common cross-border processes.

3   National Framework for EHR Systems

3.1   Overall Architectural Model

The national framework of EHR in Italy is a system of systems composed by all the regional interoperabile EHR systems able to share health documents by providing and using a set of health services. Each regional EHR system is been developing (or will be developed) in accordance with the requirements specified by the norm, guidelines and specifications. The defined framework allows the preservation of the various regional EHR systems autonomy, and enables interoperability between them. The architecture of each system is characterized by: (i) a central registry for the management of metadata associated to the health documents related to patients for the localization and management of these ones, and (ii) health repositories containing clinical documents. Each patient has a single reference region, called Healthcare Assistance Region (RDA). The Healthcare Assistance Region has to manage all the documents related to its patients, not only those produced in its healthcare facilities, but also the documents created in another region. In the case a patient is cured in a region different from RDA after having required a health care service, the clinical document produced is archived in a repository of this region, which is in charge of providing metadata about the document to the Healthcare Assistance Region. For this reason, the regional systems expose a set of services, including: search for documents, retrieve documents, communicate metadata to RDA.

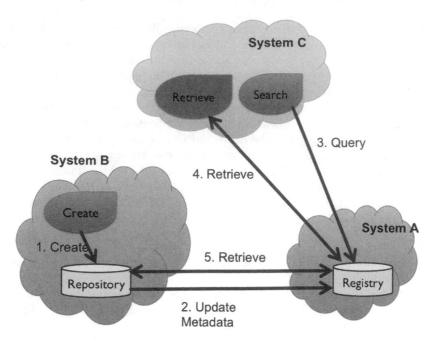

Fig. 1. Interactions among the regional EHR systems.

Figure 1 shows the interactions between three possible regional EHR systems:

- creation of a clinical document (operations 1. Create and 2. Update Meta-data);
- search for and retrieve a clinical document (operations 3. Query and 4. Retrieve).

The interaction for the creation of a clinical document expects that a patient (with RDA = System A) points to system B for a clinical event. In this way, the system B generates a document, which is inserted in a repository. Then the system B sends the metadata of the document to system A. The search and retrieve interactions require that the system C searches for the document (created before). The patient's RDA system is represented by the system A, so the search operation is carried out from the system A, after that system C requests to retrieve the document to the system A, which finally requests it to the system B and manages the request acting as a proxy. It is clear that these iterations require the knowledge of a range of information, including for example the patient's RDA. Below in paragraph Sect. 3.3 the processes related to these interactions are detailed.

3.2   Requirements of EHRs

Several organizational and architectural constraints are taken into account in the definition of the architecture for the interoperability framework for EHR systems. The main constraints are the following:

- **Patient Consent:** every patient can take advantage of the functionalities offered by the EHR system of the health care provider region of the patient. To this aim, she/he has to express two types of consent: (i) Uploading consent, which is a consent enabling the population of the EHR with her/his clinical documents by the health facilities; (ii) Consultation consent, which is a consent enabling the consultation of the EHR by health professionals. Specifically, the patient is allowed choosing the professional roles permitted to access her/his EHR by defining specific privacy policies.
- **Index Metadata Model:** the Healthcare Assistance Region of the patient has the responsibility of maintaining index metadata related to all the documents related to its patients, even if such documents are produced and maintained by health facilities sited outside the region.
- **Proxy-based Interoperability Model:** the system of the health care provider region has to operate as a mediator with the other regional systems in all the cross-border processes in which its patients are involved.
- **First Implementation of EHRs:** even if EHRs can contain a multitude of topologies of information, the first mandatory kinds of clinical documents to be accessible via EHR are patient summary and laboratory report. Then, in the first phase, only details about the finality of care of the patient are defined.

3.3   Cross-Border Processes

This subsection describes the set of cross-border processes that have been defined in order to enable the application communication among regional EHR systems.

The interoperability requirement among EHR systems requests a shared architecture topology at national level, for which each regional EHR system must provide a set of interoperability services.

All the regional nodes cooperate according to a joint architectural model based on a federated approach, by exposing and invoking the services of the other nodes. These services are needed for sharing all EHR information at national level. Each regional node has to offer a series of services designed to ensure interoperability with other regional nodes, which themselves make use of these services. In the context of interregional interactions, such nodes can be grouped in three classes:

- **Provider Node:** is the node that offers an interoperability services.
- **Consumer Node:** is the node that benefits from an interoperability service.
- **Proxy Node:** is a node that provides support services.

The interactions among different types of nodes are shown in Fig. 2.

Every regional EHR systems have to implement cross-border processes (and the related services) according to a Service Oriented Architecture (SOA) paradigm. Such processes have to satisfy a set of national business processes, according to which each region may assume a different role (Fig. 3):

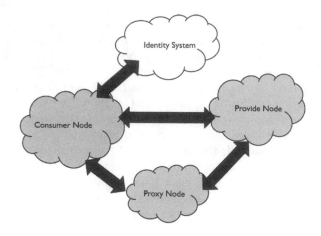

Fig. 2. Interactions among nodes.

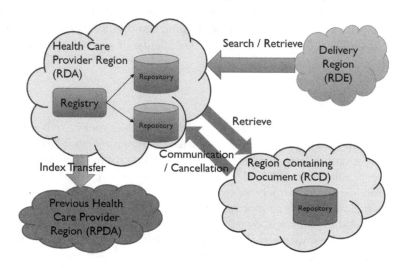

Fig. 3. Roles in the cross-border processes.

- **RDA** (Healthcare Assistance Region): is the region that manages (through metadata) clinical documents and security policies related to a patient which the region has in charge. The document management is performed by memorizing specific metadata associated to documents, allowing thus the localization and management of the clinical resources;
- **RCD** (Region Containing a Document): is the region in which a specific document has been created and maintained; the document is stored in a repository of the region, but the metadata are managed by RDA (RCD can coincide also with RDA);

- **RDE** (Region of Service Delivery): is the region that provides an health service to a patient, so RDE is able to search for a document and/or to create a document;
- **RPDA** (Previous Healthcare Assistance Region): is the region that previously has taken in charge a patient, managing his/her clinical documents. The patient may choose to change his/her Healthcare Assistance Region: in this case all the metadata and policies will have to be transferred from RPDA to the new RDA.

The possible cross-border processes are described below:

- *Searching for documents*: RDE requires RDA to consult the EHR of the patient. RDA returns the list of documents for which the user has access rights. Figure 4a shows the request of this service.
- *Retrieving a document*: RDE, after obtaining the list of documents, requires RDA retrieving a document. RDA returns the document if the user has access rights. Eventually, RDA forwards the request to RCD if the document is available outside. Figure 4b shows the request of this service.
- *Creating or updating a document*: RDE transmits to RDA the list of metadata of a document created/updated for a patient of this one (the document is stored in RDE, which therefore serves as RCD). RDA stores the metadata in its system.
- *Invalidating a document*: RCD requires RDA to perform a logical deletion of metadata related to a document, due to the invalidation of this one.
- *Transferring of index*: a new RDA requires RPDA to transfer the index of the EHR (list of all metadata and privacy policies) associated with the patient. RPDA returns the index, which is registered in the new RDA, and then disable it. After the transfer, the invalidation process on the transfered documents has to be performed.
- *Patient identification*: RDE requires the Identity System, which is a central system at the national level, the identification of a patient, in order to obtain the patient's personal data (such as name, surname, etc.) and a patient identification assertion. Figure 4a shows the request of this service.

Figure 4 shows the relationship between regional systems through the processes. In order to achieve semantic interoperability, several standards in different domains exists, e.g. CIDOC-CRM [10] in the cultural domain. Due to its specificity, to assure semantic interoperability for the e-health domain, suitable standards have been individuated: HL7 CDA Rel. 2 specifies the structure and semantics of clinical documents, whereas clinical content is represented by using a set of classification and coding systems, like the international standards International Classification of Diseases, Ninth Revision, Clinical Modification (ICD9-CM), Logical Observation Identifiers Names and Codes (LOINC) and Anatomical Therapeutic Chemical (ATC) or the national standard Marketing Authorization (AIC).

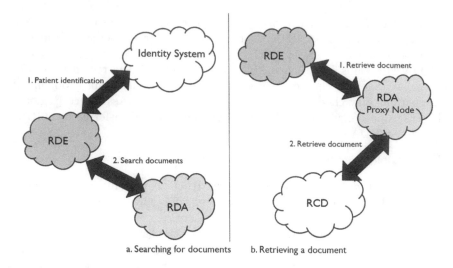

a. Searching for documents   b. Retrieving a document

Fig. 4. Roles in the cross-border processes.

4 Technical Details

4.1 Architecture Components of EHR Systems

All the regional EHR systems are based on the registry/repository paradigm. The clinical documents produced by the health facilities are stored in repositories and indexed in a regional registry (managed by RDA) by means of appropriate metadata. The metadata, as mentioned above, are appropriate information associated with the document that allow the management of the documents, including the ability to locate them. For each clinical document is necessary to manage a set of metadata. The mandatory metadata are: document type, document state, document identifier, creation date, author identifier, patient identifier, repository reference. The interoperability of the regional EHR systems is based on a nationwide federated model, based on a System-of-Systems approach, where each regional system is realized by taking into account local needs. In order to make the regional systems able to interoperate each other, each EHR system exposes a set of cross-border services, which preliminarly verify the possession of the rights by the user and provide all the functionalities needed to manage, search, and consult metadata and documents. The architecture of the distributed system at national level is shown in Fig. 5.

The security model adopted is based on a Circle of Trust among the regions. Each region is responsible for the claims made in the process of request of the cross-border services provided by the other regions. In addition, all the communications among the regional systems are exchanged through the Public Connectivity System (SPC), the Italian technological infrastructure for exchanging information assets and data between Public Administrations. Specifically, every

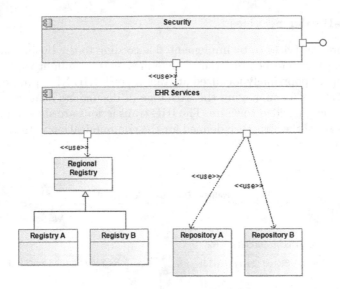

Fig. 5. Architecture of a regional EHR system.

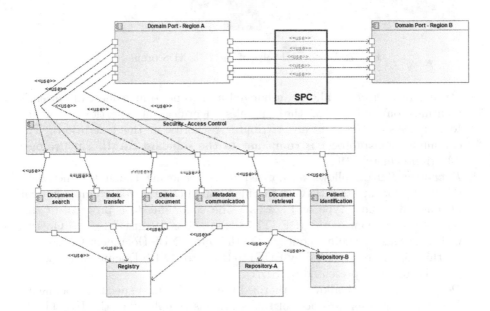

Fig. 6. Interactions among EHR systems through the SPC infrastructure.

cross-border service is linked to the SPC infrastructure by means of specific software components called Domain Ports, as shown in Fig. 6.

4.2   Cross-Border Services

The cross-border services to be implemented according to the business processes described above have to be able to exchange messages compliant to IHE XDS.b transactions [6], opportunely localized at Italian level. IHE XDS profile [11] provides specifications for managing the exchange of documents that care delivery organizations have decided to share. The IHE transactions are shown in Fig. 7. A brief description of the structure defined for the communication with the services is provided below:

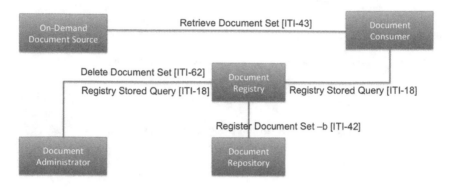

Fig. 7. Actors and roles of the IHE XDS profile.

1. *Patient Identification*: allows authorized user to perform request of patient's identification and obtain the patient's identification assertion from the Identity System (that is an Attribute Authority in the federation). The communication protocol is compliant to the standard SAML 2.0 Protocol "AttributeQuery" [16].
2. *Document Search*: allows authorized users retrieving the index metadata related to documents satisfying specified search criteria (for example patient id, date, document type and status). The communication protocol of this service is compliant to the IHE ITI-18 transaction (Registry Stored Query), which consists in sending a query from the actor "XDS Document Consumer" (in this context represented by RDE) to the actor "XDS Document Registry" (in this context represented by RDA).
3. *Document Retrieval*: allows authorized users retrieving a specified document. The communication protocol of this service is compliant to the IHE ITI-43 transaction (Retrieve Document Set), which enables the request for document retrieval from the actor "XDS Document Consumer" (in this context RDE) to the actor "XDS Document Repository" (in this context, RDA).
4. *Metadata Communication*: allows authorized users sending index metadata to the health care assistance region of the patient to which a created/updated document refers to. The communication protocol of this service is compliant to the IHE ITI-42 transaction (Register Document Set-b), which enables

the submission of metadata from the actor "XDS Integrated Document Source/Repository" (in this context RDE = RCD) to the actor "XDS Document Registry" (in this context RDA).

5. *Index Transfer*: allows transferring the index of the EHR related to a patient from a regional system to another, after the change of the health care assistence region by the patient. The communication protocol of this service is compliant to the IHE ITI-18 transaction (Registry Stored Query), which enables the actor "XDS Document Consumer" (in this context the new RDA region) to send a request to retrieve all the EHR index of a given patient to the actor "XDS Document Registry" (in this context RPDA).

6. *Delete Document*: allows authorized users the cancellation of the metadata associated with a given document. The communication protocol of this service is compliant to the ITI-62 transaction (Delete Document Set), which enables the actor "XDS Document Administrator" (in this context, in the case of invalidation of a document correponds to RCD, or, in the case of EHR index transfer to RDA) to forward the document reference to be deleted to the actor "XDS Document Registry" (in this context, in case of invalidation of a document corresponds to RDA, or, in the case of EHR index transfer to RPDA), which provides the logic deletion of the requested document.

4.3   Security Issues

The main security issues treated concern user identification and access control, in that aspects like integrity, confidentiality and auditing are assured by the use of the SPC infrastructure as a secure channel of communication among the Italian Public Administrations. With specific regard to user identification and access control, the claims to be transmitted by every region in the SOAP messages exchanged among the cross-border services are attested by digitally signed SAML 2.0 assertions.

Each regional system must provide, as described above, a set of services to allow other systems communicating each other. For this reason, the definition of a shared security model has been a necessary step. The main security requirements that must be satisfied at the regional level are:

- Consent management;
- Visibility policies and obscuration;
- Access control;
- Patient identification.

The security model adopted in the Italian context allows the protection of the services offered by the regional EHR systems and the documents they maintain, by meeting the security requirements established by the national norms. Thus, it enables to respect the patient's will expressed in terms of privacy. In fact the patient can provide or not the consents to the use of his/her EHR and he/she is able to specify who can access or not on his/her documents.

Consent Management. In Italy, the patient has to provide two different types of consents for making his/her EHR accessible, which are the "uploading" and "consultation" consents. If the patient provides the uploading consent, he/she allows healthcare professionals feeding the EHR with the clinical documents produced by them. Instead, with the consultation consent, he/she enables health professionals to access his/her clinical documents. The model provides the management of consents through meta-information stored in the patient's RDA. The meta-information about the consents are used both when creating a new document (in this case the uploading consent is verified) and when research documents (in this case the consultation consent is verified).

Patient Identification. A healthcare professional who intends to access a EHR has preliminarily to identify the patient of interest, because he/she has to be sure that the clinical information that she/he is going to receive in response is related to the patient for who she/he is carrying out a health service. This phase allows identifying the patient starting from his/her identification (the Italian fiscal code) or other personal information, such as name, surname and date of birth. This solution requires the presence of a national centralized Master Patient Index (MPI), and an appropriate service, named Identity Service. This service, received the request for identification, constructs an identity assertion, containing the information related to: current fiscal code, along with a set of possible previous fiscal codes, surname (at born), name, gender, date of birth, city of birth, province of birth, address of residence, Healthcare Assistance Region, etc. The identification assertion is included in the request messages for the provider system.

Access Control. The patient, according to the indications of the Italian Data Protection Authority, has to be able to indicate the set of healthcare professional roles that can have access to each clinical document of her/his EHR (visibility policies). The patient has also to be able to obscure (making inaccessible) her/his documents to specific healthcare professional roles (obscuration). The security model allows defining visibility policies and obscuration by managing appropriate meta-information associated with clinical documents, which precisely indicate the roles on the system that can access and the ones that cannot access for all the clinical documents. The meta-information is stored in the regional node of patient's RDA and used at the time of the request of the search for documents service. This meta-information is entered after the creation of the document, even if can be successively modified. With regards to the visibility policies and obscuration, appropriate security mechanisms based on access control techniches is used (more details are in [26]). The standard adopted for authentication and authorization data exchange is the Security Assertion Markup Language (SAML) [23]. SAML enables the exchange of assertions among different domains (different regional EHR systems), thus achieving the Single-Sign-On (SSO) among different EHR regional systems. This solution involves the use of SAML 2.0 and three different assertions: *identification assertion*, *attribute assertion*, and *RDA identity assertion*. The attribute and RDA identity assertions are built by the regional system of the healthcare professional (that is RDE). The access control approach consists in two different phases: the first phase is represented by the authentication of health professionals and patients, whereas the second one consists in the verification of the authorization for accessing clinical documents. Each system has its regional Attribute Authority (AA), which is a certification authority known at regional level. After the identification, the AA is in charge of constructing the attribute assertion. The identification assertion is built by the national centralized Identity System. All the assertions have to be digitally signed using the certificates and private keys issued by the central shared Certification Authority (CA), as better described below. During the authentication phase, the regional system has to: i) verify the user identities and the correct authentication of a healthcare professional, ii) generate the appropriate SAML assertion, which has to be sent to the provider system (another regional EHR system). The provider system must first verify the validity of the received SAML assertions (for example, the digital signatures) and then may authorize or not the healthcare professional to access its services.

Secure Message Exchange. During the exchange of clinical messages among regional EHR system, it is necessary satisfy the following requirements: *message confidentiality, message integrity, non-repudiation* of forwarded messages, *access control* of actors and services. The Web Services Security (WS-Security) [12] standard specifications are adopted and the communication can be protected by using Hyper Text Transfer Protocol over Secure Socket Layer (HTTPS), on the top of the Transport Layer Security (TLS) standard. The exchanged SOAP messages have to contain the SAML assertions defined above, which are evaluated before being passed to the web service in charge. A portfolio of security assertions must be contained in all the transmitted messages. This portfolio contains the identity of the user who wants to access the EHR services, the user attributes (i.e. the user's role), information such as the purpose of use, the context in which the user is operating (e.g. ordinary or emergency), etc. The identity management is performed through a Circle of Trust of all the regional systems, which permits mutual trust relationships between the domains. In this way, the identity of the actors involved in the supra-regional transactions is ensured by a central trusted authority, which issues digital certificates to the regional domains. The message integrity is guaranteed by the use of the digital signature, which, along with the encryption, assures the non-repudiation of the forwarded messages. It is worth noting that some of these requirements are satisfied by the underlying SPC technological infrastructure. A more detailed description of the different kind of SAML assertions is reported below:

- *Identification Assertion*: certifies the identification data of a patient and her/his Healthcare Assistance Region; the assertion is issued by the national Identity System.
- *Attribute Assertion*: certifies the data relating to the user making the request, the operating environment and the type of activities to perform; the assertion is issued by the region that intends to use a cross-border service offered by another region.

– *RDA Identity Assertion*: certifies the identity of the Healthcare Assistance Region of the patient (RDA). This assertion, issued by RDA, is used in case of a request sent by RDE for retrieving a document available in RCD, through RDA, which acts as a proxy. RCD uses this assertion to verify if the request is really sent by RDA.

4.4   Central Services

In order to support the cooperation among the EHR systems, a national technical platform providing a set of central services has been realized. The services implemented have been identified analyzing the needs indicated by the regions in their project plans for the realization of their EHR systems.

The purposes of these services vary from managing service endpoints, to enabling the homogeneous presentation of the clinical documents represented according to the XML-based HL7 CDA format by means of national style sheets, to handling the terminologies. Besides, in order to support the correct development of the cross-border services by the regions, a test environment realizing the business processes described above has been implemented.

Such a test environment is able to simulate the behavior of a typical regional EHR system and allows regional domains verifying the correctness of the request

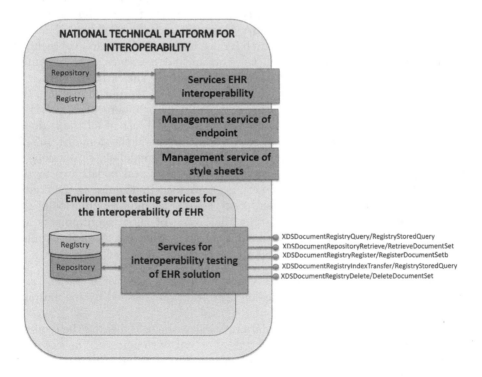

Fig. 8. National platform for EHR interoperability.

messages for the invocation of the cross-border services. The set of interoperability services have been developed and made available in the national platform, as shown in Fig. 8. The developed platform provides in particular a test environment that allow the simulation of the interoperability services in accordance with the defined specifications: in this way the regions can simulate and test the request messages and identify the correct responses of the interoperability services. In order to enable this phase of testing, a Circle of Trust based on a single Certification Authority, which provides and maintains digital certificates used for digital signatures of the security assertions, has been set up.

5   Conclusions

In this paper, the Italian technological framework for EHR interoperability defined from a National Technical Board was presented. The architectural model of the framework was formalized in order to make interoperable the EHR systems developed by the Italian regions each other, preserving the privacy of the patients. The framework meets the organizational, functional and technical requirements provided by the Italian norms on EHR. In this scenario, patients clinical documents are accessible to all the authorized health professionals regardless of the region where the patient benefits from medical care. In order to ensure the privacy, the patient has to provide two different types of consents for making his EHR accessible, which are the "uploading" and "consultation" consents. In addition, the patient is able to define specific visibility policies, allowing or denying the access to her/his clinical documents on the basis on health professional roles. The availability of the documents is guaranteed by cross-border services based on the IHE XDS profile, which every regional EHR system has to make available, according to national common cross-border business processes. The security model of the national framework is based on the adoption of specific security standards, such as WS-Security and SAML assertions, which contain information about patient, health professional, context of use. SAML assertions are transmitted by every region in the SOAP messages exchanged among the cross-border services, in order to enable the verification of the access rights to EHR resources. Therefore, some central services have made available, including in particular a test environment that allow the simulation of the interoperability services in accordance with the national technical specifications. In this way, the regions can simulate and test the request messages and identify the correct responses of the interoperability services. As future work, it is planned to specify further technical details about some relevant aspects, like homogeneous use of digital signatures, style sheets, user access, coding systems and consent obtainment. These technical details will be addressed within interregional working groups.

Acknowledgements. The work presented in this paper has been partially supported by two joint projects between the Agency for Digital Italy and the National Research Council of Italy: Interventions to support the realization of the Electronic Health Record, prot. CNR 25751/2014, and Realization of services of the national interoperability infrastructure for the Electronic Health Record, det. AgID 61/2015.

References

1. (2016). http://www.istat.it/it/files/2015/09/Dimensioni-salute.pdf
2. (2016). http://www.en13606.org/
3. (2016). http://www.hl7.org/
4. (2016). http://hl7.org/fhir/summary.html
5. (2016). http://openehr.org/
6. (2016). http://www.ihe.net/
7. (2016). https://www.infoway-inforoute.ca/en/
8. (2016). http://sequoiaproject.org/ehealth-exchange/
9. (2016). http://www.epsos.eu/
10. (2016). http://www.cidoc-crm.org/official_release_cidoc.html
11. (2016). http://wiki.ihe.net/index.php/Cross-Enterprise_Document_Sharing
12. (2016). https://www.oasis-open.org/committees/tc_home.php?wg_abbrev=wss
13. Aminpour, F., Sadoughi, F., Ahamdi, M.: Utilization of open source electronic health record around the world: a systematic review. Off. J. Isfahan Univ. Med. Sci. **19**(1), 57–64 (2014)
14. Beale, T.: Archetypes: constraint-based domain models for future-proof information systems. In: OOPSLA 2002 Workshop on Behavioural Semantics, vol. 105 (2002)
15. Black, A.D., Car, J., Pagliari, C., Anandan, C., Cresswell, K., Bokun, T., McKinstry, B., Procter, R., Majeed, A., Sheikh, A.: The impact of ehealth on the quality and safety of health care: a systematic overview. PLOS Med. **8**(1), 1–16 (2011)
16. Cantor, S., Kemp, I.J., Philpott, N.R., Maler, E.: Assertions and protocols for the oasis security assertion markup language v2.0. OASIS Standard (2005), March 2005 http://wiki.ihe.net/index.php/Cross-Enterprise_Document_Sharing
17. Chiaravalloti, M., Ciampi, M., Pasceri, E., Sicuranza, M., De Pietro, G., Guarasci, R.: A model for realizing interoperable EHR systems in Italy. In: International HL7 Interoperability Conference Proceedings, pp. 13–22. HL7 Conference 2015 (2015). http://ihic2015.hl7cr.eu/Proceedings-web.pdf
18. Ciampi, M., Esposito, A., Guarasci, R., De Pietro, G.: Towards interoperability of EHR systems: the case of Italy. In: Proceedings of the International Conference on Information and Communication Technologies for Ageing Well and e-Health, vol. 1, pp. 133–138. ICT4AWE (2016)
19. Ciampi, M., Pietro, G., Esposito, C., Sicuranza, M., Mori, P., Gebrehiwot, A., Donzelli, P.: On securing communications among federated health information systems. In: Ortmeier, F., Daniel, P. (eds.) SAFECOMP 2012. LNCS, vol. 7613, pp. 235–246. Springer, Heidelberg (2012). doi:10.1007/978-3-642-33675-1_21
20. Dogac, A., Laleci, G.B., Aden, T., Eichelberg, M.: Enhancing IHE XDS for federated clinical affinity domain support. IEEE Trans. Inf. Technol. Biomed. **11**(2), 213–221 (2007)

21. Commission of the European Communities, E.C: Together for health: a strategic approach for the EU 2008–2013 (2007). http://ec.europa.eu/health/ph_overview/Documents/strategy_wp_en.pdf
22. Kalra, D., Blobel, B.: Semantic interoperability of EHR systems. Stud. Health Technol. Inf. **127**, 231 (2007)
23. Lawrence, K., Sun, R.M., Nadalin, A., VeriSign, P.H.B.: Web services security: saml token profile 1.1. Terminology 5(3Usage), p. 7 (2002). https://www.oasis-open.org/committees/download.php/16768/wss-v1.1-spec-os-SAMLTokenProfile.pdf
24. Ludwick, D.A., Doucette, J.: Adopting electronic medical records in primary care: lessons learned from health information systems implementation experience in seven countries. Int. J. Med. Inf. **78**(1), 22–31 (2009)
25. Shekelle, P., Morton, S.C., Keeler, E.B.: Costs and benefits of health information technology (2006)
26. Sicuranza, M., Esposito, A.: An access control model for easy management of patient privacy in EHR systems. In: 2013 8th International Conference for Internet Technology and Secured Transactions (ICITST), pp. 463–470. IEEE (2013)

Human Daily Activity and Fall Recognition Using a Smartphone's Acceleration Sensor

Charikleia Chatzaki[1,2(✉)], Matthew Pediaditis[1,2], George Vavoulas[1], and Manolis Tsiknakis[1,2]

[1] Department of Informatics Engineering,
Biomedical Informatics and eHealth Laboratory,
Technological Educational Institute of Crete, Estavromenos,
71004 Heraklion, Crete, Greece
chatzaki.roula@gmail.com,
matthew.pediaditis@gmail.com, gvavoo@gmail.com,
tsiknaki@staff.teicrete.gr
[2] Computational BioMedicine Laboratory,
Foundation for Research and Technology – Hellas,
Institute of Computer Science, Vassilika Vouton,
71110 Heraklion, Crete, Greece

Abstract. As one of the fastest spreading technologies and due to their rich sensing features, smartphones have become popular elements of modern human activity recognition systems. Besides activity recognition, smartphones have also been employed with success in fall detection/recognition systems, although a combined approach has not been evaluated yet. This article presents the results of a comprehensive evaluation of using a smartphone's acceleration sensor for human activity and fall recognition, including 12 different types of activities of daily living (ADLs) and 4 different types of falls, recorded from 66 subjects in the context of creating "MobiAct", a publicly available dataset for benchmarking and developing human activity and fall recognition systems. An optimized feature selection and classification scheme is proposed for each, a basic, i.e. recognition of 6 common ADLs only (99.9% accuracy), and a more complex human activity recognition task that includes all 12 ADLs and 4 falls (96.8% accuracy).

Keywords: Human activity recognition · Activities of daily living · Falls · Smartphone · Accelerometer · Dataset

1 Introduction

Human activity recognition (HAR) is the process of identifying and recognizing the activities and goals of one or more humans from an observed series of actions. In recent years, human activity recognition has evoked notable scientific interest due to its frequent use in surveillance, home health monitoring, human-computer interaction, ubiquitous health care, as well as in proactive computing. Human activities can be further decomposed as a set of basic and complex activities, namely activities of daily living (ADLs) and instrumental activities of daily living (IADLs). Typical approaches for their recognition through automated means use vision sensors, inertial sensors or a

© Springer International Publishing AG 2017
C. Röcker et al. (Eds.): ICT4AWE 2016, CCIS 736, pp. 100–118, 2017.
DOI: 10.1007/978-3-319-62704-5_7

combination of both. Exploiting the increasing tendency of smartphone users, latest published studies introduce systems which use smartphone sensors to recognize human activities [1–5]. Besides the aforementioned normal daily activities, occasionally abnormal activities may also occur. Falls can be categorized as abnormal and sudden activities of a person's physical activity routine. Thus, the detection and recognition of falls is crucial in an activity recognition system especially when this is applied for the monitoring of elders [6]. Several approaches have been published using both threshold based and machine learning techniques, with the second one outperforming in terms of recognition accuracy [7].

The aim of this work is to present an optimized system in terms of feature selection and classification for the recognition of ADLs and falls based on smartphone's triaxial accelerometer data. To this end, the open, benchmark dataset "MobiAct" [1] was further extended in the context of this study. The introduced extended version of the MobiAct dataset contains records of the accelerometer, gyroscope and orientation sensors of a smartphone from sixty six subjects in total performing twelve different types of ADLs, four different types of falls and a scenario of daily living. In order to achieve an optimized recognition system for activity and fall recognition, special emphasis was placed on the selection of the most effective features from feature sets already validated in previous published studies [1, 7, 8]. A comparison study was performed to evaluate a proposed version of a feature set optimized for basic activity recognition tasks with the MobiAct dataset, as well as with an additional dataset, with results showing higher classification accuracies than previous reported studies. Furthermore, a second feature set was elaborated and tested in a more complex activity and fall recognition task, utilizing the full capabilities provided by the diversity and richness of the MobiAct dataset.

2 Related Work

2.1 Activity Recognition

A smartphone-based recognition system is proposed in [9], in which the application of a low-pass filter and a combination of Multilayer Perceptron, LogitBoost and Support Vector Machine (SVM) classifiers reached an overall accuracy of 91.15% when the smartphone was held in the hand of the user. Samples were recorded from four volunteers while performing six activities: slow and fast running, walking, aerobic dance, ascending stairs ("stairs up") and descending stairs ("stairs down"). The sampling rate was set at 100 Hz while a window of 1.28 s with 50% overlap was used for feature extraction.

Anjum and Ilyas [10] introduced a similar approach with ten users performing seven different activities which included walking, running, stairs up, stairs down, cycling, driving and remaining inactive, by carrying the smartphone in various positions. A sampling rate of 15 Hz and matching time windows of 5 s were used. Based on the ranking of the information gain, nine features were selected from the auto correlation function. For the classification process Naïve Bayes, C4.5 Decision Tree, K-Nearest Neighbor and SVM classifiers were tested. The C4.5 Decision Tree performed better than the other classifiers with an accuracy of 95.2%.

Zheng et al. [7] proposed a two-phase method to achieve recognition of four different types of activities (sitting, standing, walking and running) using tri-axial acceleration data from a Samsung galaxy SIII smartphone. Five subjects performed the activities with the phone placed loosely in a pocket. Records of two minutes were used for the training phase while for the testing phase data from continuous records of several days were used. A sampling rate of 100 Hz was used. In order to achieve noise reduction, the authors deployed Independent Components Analysis, specifically the fast ICA algorithm, in combination with the wavelet transform for feature extraction. For the classification, a Support Vector Machine was employed using the WEKA toolkit. A maximum accuracy of 98.78% was reported for a leave-one-out validation.

Based on tri-axial accelerometer data of a smartphone, Buber and Guvensan [11] developed a recognition system for the following activities: walking, jogging, jumping, stairs up, stairs down, sitting, standing and biking. Five volunteers performed those activities with the smartphone placed in the front pocket of their trousers. The sampling rate was set at 20 Hz and a 10 s moving window was used for feature extraction. The evaluation was performed with two feature selection algorithms (OneRAttributeEval and ReliefF AttributeEval) and six classification algorithms (J48, K-Star, Bayes Net, Naïve Bayes, Random Forest, and k-NN) using 10-fold cross-validation. The authors resulted in a combination of 15 features with k-NN to perform best at a recognition rate of 94%.

Fan et al. [12] studied three different decision tree models based on (a) the activity performed by the user and the position of the smartphone (vector), (b) only the position and (c) only the activity. Fifteen users performed five kinds of activities: stationary, walking, running, stairs up and stairs down with the smartphone placed into a carrying bag, a trouser pocket or in the hand. Ten-second samples of accelerometer data were recorded for each different kind of activity and position of smartphone. The authors concluded that the model based only on the activity outperformed the other two with an accuracy of 88.32%.

In another study [13], accelerometer data from a smartphone were recorded with a sampling frequency of 40 Hz while seven volunteers were performing five different activities: walking, running, cycling, driving a car, and sitting/standing. In each recording, four smartphones were placed in various positions, namely, trousers' front pocket, jacket's pocket, at backpack, at brachium and one was held at the ear only when it was physically allowed. For feature extraction a sliding window of 7.5 s with 25% overlap in an online (on device) application and one with 50% overlap in an offline application, were used. Classification was achieved using five classifiers based on quadratic discriminant analysis arranged in a three stage decision tree topology. Average recognition rate of almost 98.9% was reported in the offline and 90% in the online system.

Exploiting the accelerometer sensor of a smartphone [14] developed a system for recognizing simple (biking, stairs up, driving, lying, running, sitting, standing and walking) and complex (cooking, cleaning etc.) activities performed by ten participants. The sampling frequency was set at 80 Hz maximum although variations in the sampling rate were reported. Multiple windows sizes of 1, 2, 4, 8 and 16 s with 50% overlap were used. The placement of the smartphone, in terms of position and orientation, was left at each user's will. Although complex activities were classified with an accuracy of 50%, simple activities were classified with 93% accuracy with a Multilayer Perceptron and a window size of 2 s.

Saputri et al. [15] proposed a system for activity recognition in which twenty-seven subjects performed six types of activities, namely, walking, jogging, running, stairs up, stairs down and hopping. The smartphone was placed in the front trouser pocket using a sampling rate of 50 Hz. In the feature extraction process, the window size was set at 2 s, while feature selection was performed using a self-devised three-staged genetic algorithm. The use of an Artificial Neural Network produced 93% accuracy in the activity recognition.

Another activity recognition system based on smartphone sensors is proposed by Hung et al. [16] using an open dataset [17, 18], which includes six activities (standing, walking, running, upstairs, downstairs, laying) performed by thirty volunteers with the smartphone positioned at the waist. In the referred dataset, data was collected with a sampling rate of 50 Hz and pre-processing included a sliding window of 2.56 s in duration with 50% overlap. Forty-five features were extracted and three different classifies were tested, namely, Decision Tree (J48), Support Vector Machine and Logistic Regression, with the last one outperforming the others with an overall accuracy of 96%.

A comparative study exploiting the accelerometer and gyroscope sensors of a smartphone for human activity recognition was reported by Wang et al. in [19]. Using an open dataset [18] the authors introduced a feature selection method that takes advantages of filter and wrapper methods in order to conclude to a set of discriminant features. The best results, 87.8% classification accuracy, reported with the use of kNN classifier and a subset of 66 features.

2.2 Fall Detection and Recognition

Techniques to detect and automatically classify a fall, using acceleration data from a smartphone, were demonstrated in [21]. Ten second episodes with the falls and "fall-like" (uncontrolled) events positioned in the center of the episodes were created and linearly interpolated to a sampling frequency of 20 Hz. Five different classifiers were tested: SVM, Regularized Logistic Regression (RLR), Naïve Bayes, k-NN, and Decision Trees. In the testing process, 10-fold cross-validation and subject-wise cross-validation were performed.

A smartphone-based fall detection system called "FallAlarm" was introduced by Zhao et al. [22]. The investigated activities were: stationary, walking and running while the falls were: forward fall, backward fall, left fall and right fall. In their method, the acceleration signals were evaluated via a decision tree model, which performed better in comparison to Naïve Bayes and SVM classifiers. A4 s window with 50% overlap was applied.

Kansiz et al. [23] developed a fall detection system using a smartphone's accelerometer data. The activities of daily living included walking, jogging, jumping, sitting, standing, stairs up and stairs down, while the tested falls were forward fall, backward fall, side fall, hard fall and soft fall. The sampling rate was set at 20 Hz. For feature extraction a time window of 3 s in duration was applied. For the classification process, K-Star, Decision Tree and Naive Bayes classifiers were chosen. The authors report that K-star outperformed the others in a 10-fold cross-validation.

Figueiredo et al. [24] proposed a simple threshold based technique for the detection of falls. The results indicated 100% sensitivity and 93% specificity using the accelerometer data of two participants performing falls and six participants performing ADLs. Furthermore an SVM classifier was deployed and resulted on 96.16% accuracy using 3 features and 2-fold cross-validation as an evaluation method.

2.3 Summarizing Findings of Related Work

The above non-exhaustive review on activity and fall recognition systems using smartphone embedded inertial sensors reveals that several research studies have already been published, reporting acceptable results while employing various different data processing and analysis approaches. However, there is an inherent weakness of conducting objective comparisons between different implementations, because of the

Table 1. Overview of the methodologies and their results followed by the related studies for activity recognition. Partially reproduced from [1].

Study	No of subjects	Activities[a]	Sampling Frequency	Window size/overlap	No of Features	Smartphone position	Algorithms[b]	Performance
[9]	4	ADN, STN, STU, SWL FWL, RUN	100 Hz	1.28 s/50%	18	hand of the user	BN, k-Star, kNN, NB, RF, J48	MLP & LB &SVM: 91.15% Accuracy
[10]	10	BIK, DRI, INA, STC, STN, STU, RUN	15 Hz	5 s	9[c]	various positions	C4.5, kNN, SVM, NB	C4.5: 95.2%.
[20]	5	RUN, STD, WAL, SIT	100 Hz	–	ICA + Wavelet	freely in pocket	SVM	98.78%
[11]	5	BIK, JOG, JUM, SIT, STN, STU, WAL	20 Hz	10 s	15	front pocket	BN, J48, K-Star, kNN, NB, RF	k-NN: 94%
[12]	15	RUN, STU, WAL, STC, STN	–	10 s	10[c]	bag, trouser pocket & hands	ID3 DC	80.29%
[13]	7	BIK, DRI, RUN, SIT, STD, WAL	40 Hz	7.5 s/25% online app 7.5 s/50% offline app	76	5 smartphones: various position	DC & QDA	90% online 98.9% offline
[14]	10	BIK, DRI, LYI, RUN, SIT, STD, STU, WAL	80 Hz	1,2,4,8,16/50%	6	user's choice (position & orientation)	B-FT, BN, DT, K-star, MLP, NB	MLP: 93% 2 s window
[15]	27	HOP, RUN, STN, STU, WAL.	50 Hz	2 s	21	front pocket	ANN	93%
[16]	30	LYI, RUN, STD, STN, STU, WAL	50 Hz	2.56 s/50%	45	Waist	J48, LR, SVM	LR 96%
[19]	30 from [18]	LYI, SIT, STN, STU, STD, WAL	50 Hz	2.56 s/50%	74: NB, 66:kNN	Waist	kNN, NB	NB 90,1%, kNN 97,8%

[a]ADN Aerobic dancing, BIK Biking, DRI Driving, HOP Hopping, INA Inactivity, JOG Jogging, JUM Jumping, LYI Laying, RUN Running, SIT Sitting, STC Static, STD Standing, STN Stairs down, STU Stairs up, SWL slow WAL, FWL fast WAL, WALWalking.
[b]ANN Artificial neural network, B-FT Best-First Tree, BN Bayes Net, C4 5 Decision Tree, DC Decision Tree, DT Decision Table, ID3 Decision Tree, J48 Weka implementation of C4.5 DC, K-star, kNN k-Nearest Neighbors, LR Logistic Regression, MLP Multilayer Perceptron, NB Naïve Bayes, QDA Quadratic discriminant analysis, RF Random Forest, SVM Support Vector Machines.
[c]Feature set includes that number of features but is not limited to.

Table 2. Overview of the methodology and results, followed by the related studies for fall detection and recognition.

Study	No of subjects	Activities	Sampling Frequency	Window size/overlap	No of Features	Smartphone position	Algorithms[2]	Performance
[21]	15	Fall like events, 4 ADLs	20 Hz	10 s	178	Belt: Set position& orientation	C 4.5, k-NN, NB, RLR, SVM	RLR: Detection: 98% Classification: 99.6%
[22]	10	4 falls, 3 ADLs	32 Hz	4 s/50%	5	Waist	C 4.5, NB, SVM	C 4.5 100% Precision, 75,8% Recall
[23]	8	4 falls, 6 ADLs	20 Hz	3 s	5 to 43	Pocket	J48, k-Star, NB	K-StarAverage recall 0.88
[24]	2 falls, 6 ADLs	10 falls, 17 ADLs	50 Hz, 100 Hz	–	3	Trouser pocket, Belt	SVM, threshold algorithms	SVM 96.19%

heterogeneity of the acquired raw data, as shown in Tables 1 and 2. The issue of differentiation in smartphone positions, sampling frequency and kinds of activities and falls, along with the relatively small number of subject recordings is addressed with the use of the publicly available MobiAct dataset. Moreover, there is no constancy in the computational methodology applied for both fall detection/recognition and activity recognition, rather each task is handled separately. In this work, the proposed computational methodology (see Sect. 4.3) has been tested and evaluated in order to handle the recognition of falls and activities as a unified system.

3   The MobiAct Dataset

3.1   Dataset Description

MobiAct is a publicly available dataset (available for download from www.bmi. teicrete.gr) which includes data recorded from a smartphone's inertial sensor while participants were performing different types of activities and a range of falls. It is based on the previously released MobiFall dataset [7], which was initially created with fall detection in mind. The fact that MobiFall included various activities of daily living made it also suitable for research in human activity recognition. The latest version of MobiAct has been used in the context of this study.

The MobiAct dataset includes 4 different types of falls and 12 different ADLs from a total of 66 subjects with more than 3200 trials, all captured with a smartphone. The activities of daily living were selected based on the following criteria: (a) Activities which are fall-like were firstly included. These include sequences where the subject usually stays motionless at the end, in different positions, such as sitting on a chair or stepping in and out of a car; (b) Activities which are sudden or rapid and are similar to falls, like jumping and jogging; (c) The most common everyday activities like walking, standing, ascending and descending stairs (stairs up and stairs down). These activities were included from the start of the effort, since our ultimate objective has been to extend our original work towards recognition of not only falls, but also complex everyday activities and, eventually, behaviour patterns. Moreover, the fact that such activities are included is an advantage concerning human activity recognition in general. The latest addition to the MobiAct dataset includes two extra types of ADLs ("chair up" and "sitting"), and five different continuous sequences of daily living, which include all the different types of the separate ADLs mentioned above. These sequences of the activities are based on a scenario of daily living where a person leaves her/his home, takes her/his car to get to her/his working place (although real driving was not recorded), reaches her/his office, sits on the chair and starts working. Once she/he gets off his work, she/he takes her/his car and goes in an open area to perform physical exercise. At the end of the day she/he gets into the car and returns back home. The initial scenario was split into five sub-scenarios (continuous sequences), which are connected with idle ADLs ("standing" and "sitting"), in order to avoid recording issues that would lead to several repetitions and the frustration of the participants. The main purpose for the construction of scenarios is to investigate how the recognition of different activities with natural transitions between them in continuous recordings, will affect the performance of the system, since in a real life scenario there is no clear separation from one activity to another. This investigation is part of our ongoing work. As a result, MobiAct is suitable for investigating both fall detection/recognition and human activity recognition tasks. Tables 3 and 4 summarize all recorded activities (and activity codes), their present trial counts, durations and a short description.

Table 3. Falls recorded in the MobiAct dataset.

Code	Activity	Trials	Duration	Description
FOL	Forward-lying	3	10 s	Fall Forward from standing, use of hands to dampen fall
FKL	Front-knees-lying	3	10 s	Fall forward from standing, first impact on knees
SDL	Sideward-lying	3	10 s	Fall sideward from standing, bending legs
BSC	Back-sitting-chair	3	10 s	Fall backward while trying to sit on a chair

3.2 Dataset Acquisition Details

All activities related to the design of the acquisition protocol and the production of the MobiAct dataset itself were performed at the Technological Educational Institute of Crete. Data was recorded from the accelerometer, gyroscope and orientation sensors of a Samsung Galaxy S3 smartphone with the LSM330DLC inertial module (3D accelerometer and gyroscope). The orientation sensor is software-based and derives its data from the accelerometer and the geomagnetic field sensor. The gyroscope was calibrated prior to the recordings using the device's integrated tool. For the data acquisition, an Android application has been developed for the recording of raw data from the acceleration, the angular velocity and orientation [25]. In order to achieve the

Table 4. Activities of Daily Living Recorded in the MobiAct Dataset.

Code	Activity	Trials	Duration	Description
STD	Standing	1	5 min	Standing with subtle movements
WAL	Walking	1	5 min	Normal walking
JOG	Jogging	3	30 s	Jogging
JUM	Jumping	3	30 s	Continuous jumping
STU	Stairs up	6	10 s	Stairs up (10 stairs)
STN	Stairs down	6	10 s	Stairs down (10 stairs)
SCH	Stand to sit (sit on chair)	6	6 s	Transition from standing to sitting
SIT	Sitting on chair	1	1 min	Sitting on a chair with subtle movements
CHU	Sit to stand (chair up)	6	6 s	Transition from sitting to standing
CSI	Car step in	6	6 s	Step in a car
CSO	Car step out	6	6 s	Step out of a car
LYI	Lying	12	–	Activity taken from the lying period after a fall

highest sampling rate possible the parameter "SENSOR_DELAY FASTEST" was enabled. Finally, each sample was stored along with its timestamp in nanoseconds.

The techniques that have been applied in the majority of published studies, as presented in Sect. 2, which focus on smartphone-based activity recognition and fall detection/recognition, require the smartphone to be rigidly placed on the human body and with a specific orientation. For this purpose a strap is frequently used. In contrast to this and in an attempt to simulate every-day usage of mobile phones, our device was located in a trousers' pocket freely chosen by the subject in any random orientation. For the falls, the subjects used the pocket on the opposite side of the direction of the fall to protect the device from damage. For the simulation of falls a relatively hard mattress of 5 cm in thickness was employed to dampen the fall [7].

3.3   Dataset Participants

The MobiAct dataset currently includes records from 66 participants, 51 men and 15 women. In particular, 66 subjects performed the falls described in Table 3, 59 subjects performed nine of the eleven ADLs described in Table 4, while 19 performed all the ADLs, and finally 19 subjects performed the five sequences representing the scenario of daily living described in Sect. 3.1. The subjects' age spanned between 20 and 47 years, the height ranged from 160 cm to 193 cm, and the weight varied from 50 kg to 120 kg. The average profile of the subject that occurs based on the described characteristics is 26 years old, 176 cm of height and 76 kg weight. All participants had different physical status, ranging from completely untrained to athletes (minimum of cases). The challenge of the generalization [26] is addressed due to the high number of participants, the range of ages and the range of physical status included in the MobiAct dataset.

4 Methods

4.1 Datasets for Comparison and Evaluation

Our intention in generating MobiAct was to enable testing and benchmarking between various methods for human activity recognition with smartphones. As a result a comparison to other existing and publically available datasets is of significant value. The most suitable such public dataset is the WISDM dataset [2]. Both WISDM and MobiAct datasets include a large set of the same ADLs, namely walking, jogging, stairs up, stairs down, sitting and standing, in a common file format. Moreover, the position of the mobile device is equally treated in both datasets since it was left up to each subject to freely select the orientation of the smartphone into their pocket.

Other freely available datasets, such as the DALIAC dataset [27] and the UCI dataset [17] could not be used for comparison, since they differ significantly in terms of the recorded ADLs and the data acquisition conditions. Specifically, the DALIAC dataset uses multiple accelerometer nodes statically placed on the human body. It does not use the smartphone-based inertial sensors and therefore it is not suitable for the study at hand. The UCI data, on the other hand, was recorded with a specific position for the smartphone (waist mounted) and does not include the jogging activity, which is part of both MobiAct and WISDM datasets, but instead includes the lying down activity, which is not part of MobiAct and WISDM. Apart from these differences, significant differences in the data format prevented the utilization of the UCI dataset.

4.2 Reproduction of the WISDM Study

An important qualitative part of this investigation is the validation of the feature extraction techniques through the reproduction of a published computational pipeline and the comparison of the results. For this purpose the reported study from Kwapisz et al. [2] was selected, which uses the WISDM dataset. Our hypothesis is that, if the results of our reproduction of the WISDM study are approximately the same as the published results, then the feature set defined could be used for a comparison to other feature sets, such as the one reported by Vavoulas et al. [7]. For this comparison a subset of MobiAct was used. Specifically, the scenario recordings were excluded, since the WISDM does not include comparable data.

In order to extract features from the two selected datasets a common file format and sampling rate for both had to be achieved. Following MobiAct's file format, the WISDM raw data file was split into smaller files based on the subject's ID and activity. Linear interpolation and subsampling was applied on the MobiAct data in order to achieve a 20 Hz sampling frequency which is what is used for the production of the WISDM dataset. 20 Hz as a sampling frequency is also reported by Shoaib et al. [28] as being suitable for the recognition of ADLs from inertial sensors. In MobiAct, the duration of some types of activities was smaller than 10 s, which is the time window for feature extraction that the WISDM study uses [2]. To achieve a minimum of 10 s trial duration especially in trials of stairs up, stairs down and sitting the last sample of each file in question was padded.

The results of our effort to reproduce the WISDM study are presented in Table 5. In general the reproduced and the reported results have the same behaviour in both studies. Some minor deviations may be due to slight differences in the windowing and feature extraction methodology, since, as previously mentioned, we had to split the WISDM data into smaller files.

4.3   Feature Extraction and Feature Sets

In attempting to estimate the parameters for an optimized computational and analysis pipeline, it is obvious that the selection of a respective optimized feature set is of paramount importance. To construct this feature set, a combination of the features used in the study employing the precursor of MobiAct [7] and the WISDM study [2] were used.

Feature Set A(FSA)
This feature set consists of 68 features based on the reported work in [7]. For most of the features a value was extracted for each of the three axes (x, y, z). In detail, the following features were computed within each time window:

- 21 features in total from: Mean, median, standard deviation, skew, kurtosis, minimum and maximum of each axis (x, y, z) of the acceleration.
- 1 feature from: The slope SL defined as:

$$SL = \sqrt{(max_x - min_x)^2 + (max_y - min_y)^2 + (max_z - min_z)^2} \qquad (1)$$

- 4 features from: Mean, standard deviation, skew and kurtosis of the tilt angle TA_i between the gravitational vector and the y-axis (since the orientation of the smartphone was not predefined it is expected that the negative y-axis will not be always pointing towards the vertical direction). The tilt angle is defined as:

$$TA_i = \sin^{-1}\left(\frac{y_i}{\sqrt{x_i^2 + y_i^2 + z_i^2}}\right) \qquad (2)$$

where x, y and z is the acceleration in the respective axis.
- 11 features from: Mean, standard deviation, minimum, maximum, difference between maximum and minimum, entropy of the energy in 10 equal sized blocks, short time energy, spectral centroid, spectral roll off, zero crossing rate and spectral flux from the magnitude of the acceleration vector.
- 31 additional features were calculated from the absolute signals of the accelerometer, including mean, median, standard deviation, skew, kurtosis, minimum, maximum and slope.

Feature Set B (FSB)
A total of 43 features were generated in accordance to the WISDM study reported by Kwapisz et al. [2] as variants of six basic features. For each of the three axes, the

average acceleration, standard deviation, average absolute difference, time between peaks and binned distribution ($\times$ 10 bins) were calculated in addition to the average resultant acceleration as a single feature.

First Optimized Feature Set (OFS1)

Following elaborate experimentation (totally 70 different experimental setting) on the subset of 6 activities covered by both the WISDM and MobiAct datasets in which (a) various combinations of window size (10, 5, 2 s) and overlap (0%, 50%, 80%) were tested, (b) features were removed or added into the feature vector based on observations of the achieved accuracy, and (c) different classifiers were employed, such as IBk (kNN), J48, Logistic regression and Multilayer Perceptron (from the WEKA's algorithm set), a first optimized feature set has been produced. All experiments were conducted using 10-fold cross-validation. Specifically, the two feature sets (FSA and FSB), obtained using a time window of 5 s and 80% overlap, were at first combined to form one new feature set. Subsequently weak features, identified through a trial-and-error approach, were taken out in an iterative process until the best overall accuracy for both datasets (MobiAct and WISDM) was obtained as shown in Table 6. A total number of 64 features were thus retained to form the first optimized feature set. The features excluded from FSA were the kurtosis for the x, y and z axes and the spectral centroid.

Table 5. Classification results (% accuracy) in comparison to the WISDM published results (10 s window size, no overlap). Reproduced from [1].

Activity	Published results (WISDM study, FSB)			Reproduced results (FSB)			Results using the first optimized feature set (OFS1)		
	J48	LR	MLP	J48	LR	MLP	J48	LR	MLP
Walking	89.9	93.6	91.7	90.8	93.8	95.3	99.4	98.3	99.8
Jogging	96.5	98.0	98.3	98.5	98.6	99.0	99.1	99.4	99.6
Stairs up	59.3	27.5	61.5	65.5	53.2	79.3	85.2	79.5	92.5
Stairs down	55.5	12.3	44.3	55.6	49.7	69.4	87.4	77.4	91.5
Sitting	95.7	92.2	95.0	97.0	94.1	94.6	97.0	97.5	98.0
Standing	93.3	87.0	91.9	97.0	94.6	90.4	99.4	97.0	99.4
Overall	**85.1**	**78.1**	**91.7**	**88.3**	**87.5**	**92.4**	**96.7**	**94.9**	**98.2**

The features excluded from FSB were: Time between peaks, binned distribution and average absolute difference. Finally, the features from OFS1 were also calculated by using a 10 s window and no overlap as defined in the WISDM study for a final comparison to their results, as shown in Table 5.

Second Optimized Feature Set (OFS2)

The first optimized feature set was further optimized for activity recognition based on the 6 common activities included in both the WISDM and the MobiAct dataset. Since

Table 6. Classification results using the first optimized feature set (5 s window size, 80% overlap). Reproduced from [1].

Dataset/Classifier:	MobiAct/IBk		MobiAct/J48		WISDM/IBk		WISDM/J48	
Activity	TP Rate	FP Rate	TP Rate	FP Rate	TP Rate	FP Rate	TP Rate	FP Rate
Walking	1.000	0.000	1.000	0.000	1.000	0.000	0.998	0.002
Jogging	1.000	0.000	1.000	0.000	0.999	0.000	0.998	0.001
Stairs up	0.993	0.001	0.930	0.004	0.992	0.001	0.939	0.006
Stairs down	0.982	0.000	0.921	0.003	0.991	0.001	0.937	0.007
Sitting	1.000	0.000	0.999	0.000	0.999	0.000	0.996	0.000
Standing	1.000	0.000	1.000	0.000	0.999	0.000	0.996	0.000
Accuracy:	**99.88%**		**99.30%**		**99.79%**		**98.63%**	

MobiAct includes more ADLs it is important to move forward towards a recognition system including all. Some of these, such as the transition from sitting to standing, are less than 2 s in duration, a fact that has to be considered when selecting the window size for feature extraction. The importance of recognizing transition activities, which are short duration activities taking place in a sequence of normal activities, is highlighted as an open issue in the study of Reyes-Ortiz et al. [29]. In addition to this, we, also, strived to further reduce the number of features of OFS1 by removing the majority of absolute value features. The tests, briefly described in [8] were performed with three different window sizes (2, 1.5, 1 s) and four subsets of OFS1. The finally selected feature set (OFS2) consists of the following 39 features taken with a window size of 1 s and an overlap of 80%:

- 21 features in total from: Mean, median, standard deviation, skew, kurtosis, minimum and maximum of each axis (x, y, z) of the acceleration.
- 1 feature from: The slope SL (1).
- 4 features from: Mean, standard deviation, skew and kurtosis of the tilt angle TAi (2).
- 10 features from: Mean, standard deviation, minimum, maximum, difference between maximum and minimum, entropy of the energy in 10 equal sized blocks, short time energy, spectral roll off, zero crossing rate and spectral flux from the magnitude of the acceleration vector.
- 3 features from: The kurtosis of the absolute of the acceleration in each axis (x, y, z).

Using this feature set and the two best performing classifiers (IBk and J48) we performed a generalized evaluation with the total of 16 activities (falls included) from the MobiAct dataset, as opposed to the limited number of activities commonly used in the literature (cf. Sect. 2). A 10-fold cross-validation was used on both the complete MobiAct dataset, as well as on a subset that did not include the consecutive activities recorded for the daily living scenario. The intention for this was to perform a preliminary examination of the impact of using consecutive sequences of activities. The results are shown in Tables 7, 8, 9 and 10.

Table 7. Classification results using the J48 decision tree without the activities from the scenarios. Values below 0.80 are highlighted in italic.

Activity	TP Rate	FP Rate	Precision	F-Measure
Standing	0.985	0.006	0.985	0.985
Fall: Back-sitting-chair	*0.700*	*0.003*	*0.688*	*0.694*
Lying	0.985	0.001	0.983	0.984
Sitting on chair	0.957	0.002	0.952	0.954
Sit to stand	*0.466*	*0.001*	*0.481*	*0.473*
Car step in	*0.658*	*0.006*	*0.670*	*0.664*
Car step out	*0.695*	*0.006*	*0.684*	*0.689*
Fall: Front-knees-lying	*0.619*	*0.003*	*0.620*	*0.620*
Fall: Forward-lying	*0.563*	*0.003*	*0.573*	*0.568*
Jogging	0.981	0.002	0.980	0.981
Jumping	0.982	0.001	0.983	0.983
Stand to sit	*0.694*	*0.003*	*0.703*	*0.698*
Fall: Sideward-lying	*0.575*	*0.003*	*0.610*	*0.592*
Stairs down	0.876	0.005	0.874	0.875
Stairs up	0.885	0.005	0.883	0.884
Walking	1.000	0.000	1.000	1.000
Weighted Avg.	**0.954**	**0.003**	**0.953**	**0.953**
Variance	**0.032**	**0.000**	**0.030**	**0.031**

Table 8. Classification results using the IBk classifier without the activities from the scenarios. Values below 0.80 are highlighted in italic.

Activity	TP Rate	FP Rate	Precision	F-Measure
Standing	0.987	0.005	0.989	0.988
Fall: Back-sitting-chair	0.838	0.001	0.832	0.835
Lying	0.988	0.001	0.984	0.986
Sitting on chair	0.959	0.001	0.963	0.961
Sit to stand	*0.608*	*0.001*	*0.603*	*0.605*
Car step in	0.807	0.003	0.832	0.820
Car step out	0.850	0.003	0.831	0.841
Fall: Front-knees-lying	*0.747*	*0.002*	*0.766*	*0.756*
Fall: Forward-lying	*0.688*	*0.002*	*0.723*	*0.705*
Jogging	0.988	0.001	0.991	0.990
Jumping	0.992	0.000	0.996	0.994
Stand to sit	0.810	0.002	0.779	0.794
Fall: Sideward-lying	*0.721*	*0.001*	*0.803*	*0.759*
Stairs down	0.933	0.003	0.928	0.931
Stairs up	0.948	0.003	0.929	0.938
Walking	1.000	0.001	0.997	0.998
Weighted Avg.	**0.971**	**0.002**	**0.971**	**0.971**
Variance	**0.015**	**0.000**	**0.013**	**0.014**

Table 9. Classification results using the J48 decision tree with all activities, including scenarios. Values below 0.80 are highlighted in italic.

Activity	TP Rate	FP Rate	Precision	F-Measure
Standing	0.983	0.007	0.982	0.983
Fall: Back-sitting-chair	*0.704*	*0.002*	*0.707*	*0.706*
Lying	0.984	0.001	0.982	0.983
Sitting on chair	0.973	0.002	0.970	0.972
Sit to stand	*0.449*	*0.001*	*0.463*	*0.456*
Car step in	*0.640*	*0.006*	*0.651*	*0.646*
Car step out	*0.674*	*0.006*	*0.674*	*0.674*
Fall: Front-knees-lying	*0.596*	*0.002*	*0.592*	*0.594*
Fall: Forward-lying	*0.576*	*0.002*	*0.580*	*0.578*
Jogging	0.977	0.002	0.976	0.977
Jumping	0.978	0.001	0.980	0.979
Stand to sit	*0.656*	*0.003*	*0.680*	*0.668*
Fall: Sideward-lying	*0.577*	*0.002*	*0.610*	*0.593*
Stairs down	0.841	0.006	0.854	0.847
Stairs up	0.851	0.006	0.852	0.851
Walking	0.986	0.008	0.983	0.984
Weighted Avg.	**0.947**	**0.006**	**0.947**	**0.947**
Variance	**0.033**	**0.000**	**0.031**	**0.032**

Table 10. Classification results using the IBk classifier with all activities, including scenarios. Values below 0.80 are highlighted in italic.

Activity	TP Rate	FP Rate	Precision	F-Measure
Standing	0.984	0.005	0.987	0.986
Fall: Back-sitting-chair	0.832	0.001	0.832	0.832
Lying	0.987	0.001	0.984	0.986
Sitting on chair	0.977	0.002	0.977	0.977
Sit to stand	*0.592*	*0.001*	*0.588*	*0.590*
Car step in	0.802	0.003	0.831	0.816
Car step out	0.835	0.004	0.822	0.828
Fall: Front-knees-lying	*0.756*	*0.001*	*0.764*	*0.760*
Fall: Forward-lying	*0.691*	*0.001*	*0.729*	*0.709*
Jogging	0.985	0.001	0.990	0.987
Jumping	0.990	0.000	0.996	0.993
Stand to sit	*0.788*	*0.002*	*0.773*	*0.780*
Fall: Sideward-lying	*0.721*	*0.001*	*0.795*	*0.757*
Stairs down	0.913	0.003	0.922	0.917
Stairs up	0.929	0.003	0.921	0.925
Walking	0.994	0.006	0.986	0.990
Weighted Avg.	**0.968**	**0.004**	**0.968**	**0.968**
Variance	**0.015**	**0.000**	**0.014**	**0.014**

4.4   Classifiers

The classifiers selected for the final testing of the optimized feature set were the IBk (with 1 nearest neighbor), the J48 decision tree, Logistic regression and Multilayer perceptron, included in WEKA [30] with default parameters. The first two produced the best overall results, whilst the remaining two were used for a comparison to the WISDM study since their use was also reported in the specific study.

5   Results

5.1   With Respect to the First Optimized Feature Set

The first optimized feature set was produced in the context of activity recognition related to the WISDM study (6 ADLs, no scenarios and falls). The experimental results obtained using this feature set are shown in Table 6. It is worth noticing that with both classifiers the overall accuracy is close to 99% for both datasets. The best accuracy for the MobiAct dataset is obtained with the IBk classifier. IBk generally appears to have a relative better performance with 94% accuracy, a fact that has already been reported elsewhere [11]. Also, IBk performs better than J48 for the WISDM dataset as well. The weakness in accurately recognizing activities which produce similar signals, such as stairs up and stairs down is noticeable with J48. Nevertheless, IBk recognizes these activities effectively. An additional noticeable point is that IBk performs slightly better in classifying the walking activity, which has been observed to be often misclassified as a stairs up or stairs down activity.

Considering the comparison of the results when using FSB and OFS1 with the WISDM dataset, for all the classifiers used, OFS1 outperforms FSB (Table 5).

5.2   With Respect to the Second Optimized Feature Set

The second optimized feature set was produced for activity recognition [8] using all ADLs included in MobiAct and was tested using both the ADLs and the falls. The results (in Tables 7, 8, 9 and 10) show that the second optimized feature set shows an overall good performance with the highest accuracy of 97.1% (cf. Table 8), while IBk shows slightly better performance results than the decision tree and less variance in the results. The performance on the ADLs is remarkably well for all cases. The detection of the short sit to stand and stand to sit activities is not ideal but would otherwise be impossible with a larger window. The confusion matrix for the case of using IBk with all activities shown in Table 11 shows that sit to stand (CHU) is most often misclassified as stand to sit (SCH) while the opposite is not as distinct. The recognition of activities which produce similar signals, such as stairs up and stairs down, does not seem to be a problem as observed in the above results using OFS1. The correct recognition of falls is more problematic. A closer look at the Table 11 reveals that most often the front-knees-lying fall (FKL) is misclassified as forward-lying (FOL) and vice versa. The same is noticeable for the sideward-lying fall (SDL) and back-sitting-chair fall (BSC).

Table 11. Confusion matrix of the results using the IBk classifier with all activities, including scenarios, expressed in terms of the percentage of total class instances. Values in light grey show misclassifications above 5% and values in dark grey show misclassifications above 10%.

Actual:	Classified as:															
	STD	BSC	LYI	SIT	CHU	CSI	CSO	FKL	FOL	JOG	JUM	WAL	STU	SCH	SDL	STN
STD	98.43	0.04	0.01	0.01	0.06	0.17	0.30	0.05	0.10	0.03	0.02	0.26	0.22	0.05	0.05	0.21
BSC	1.86	83.16	4.33	0.00	0.00	0.19	0.04	1.90	1.94	0.00	0.00	0.00	0.91	0.00	5.21	0.46
LYI	0.02	0.36	98.70	0.01	0.00	0.01	0.00	0.30	0.26	0.00	0.00	0.00	0.01	0.00	0.31	0.02
SIT	0.05	0.00	0.01	97.71	0.15	0.84	0.48	0.00	0.00	0.00	0.00	0.00	0.00	0.77	0.00	0.00
CHU	5.81	0.00	0.00	4.05	59.15	1.85	3.35	0.00	0.00	0.09	0.00	2.64	0.18	22.80	0.00	0.09
CSI	2.16	0.01	0.00	3.13	0.56	80.19	9.45	0.00	0.01	0.07	0.01	1.68	0.19	2.47	0.00	0.07
CSO	3.18	0.01	0.00	1.62	0.73	7.30	83.48	0.03	0.00	0.03	0.00	1.36	0.17	2.02	0.01	0.07
FKL	2.62	2.02	3.17	0.00	0.00	0.09	0.05	75.57	8.95	0.00	0.00	0.00	1.65	0.00	2.80	3.08
FOL	5.56	3.88	4.08	0.00	0.00	0.05	0.00	10.66	69.10	0.00	0.00	0.00	1.43	0.00	3.62	1.63
JOG	0.12	0.00	0.00	0.00	0.01	0.05	0.03	0.00	0.00	98.50	0.28	0.78	0.10	0.01	0.00	0.11
JUM	0.06	0.00	0.00	0.00	0.00	0.00	0.00	0.00	0.00	0.69	98.97	0.16	0.05	0.00	0.00	0.05
WAL	0.13	0.00	0.00	0.00	0.01	0.05	0.05	0.00	0.00	0.04	0.00	99.37	0.17	0.03	0.00	0.14
STU	1.15	0.04	0.01	0.00	0.01	0.04	0.02	0.02	0.06	0.02	0.00	2.53	92.95	0.02	0.04	3.10
SCH	1.75	0.00	0.00	5.12	6.56	2.67	2.98	0.00	0.00	0.03	0.03	1.77	0.26	78.81	0.00	0.03
SDL	2.83	7.92	4.18	0.00	0.00	0.22	0.09	3.87	3.05	0.00	0.00	0.00	2.79	0.00	72.14	2.92
STN	1.28	0.02	0.03	0.00	0.01	0.02	0.01	0.13	0.06	0.03	0.01	2.98	4.03	0.00	0.13	91.25

6 Conclusions

The study's objective was to estimate an optimal computational and analysis pipeline which accurately recognizes ADLs and falls exploiting an extensive dataset of motion data collected from a smartphone. As a result of this investigation two optimized sets of features were extracted, the first (OFS1) showing best results in human activity recognition with two independent datasets, and the second one (OFS2) performing remarkably well in the complex task of human activity and fall recognition. These feature sets were the outcome of many tests, through a trial and error process that removed weak features.

For the first optimized feature set the kurtosis of each axis of the acceleration was removed but it has been observed that the kurtosis features of the absolute values of the acceleration in all three axes improve the performance of classification and hence were included in the first optimized feature sets. The spectral centroid is the key feature, which negatively affects the results of activity recognition. The stairs up and stairs down activities exhibit the worst accuracy among all activities. This observation is also seen in other reports and may be related with the random device orientation or the dynamic and temporal resolution of the accelerometer sensor. The best overall accuracy in 6-class human activity recognition of 99.88% is achieved when using the IBk classification algorithm on the MobiAct dataset in combination with OFS1. This is the best reported classification result to date, when comparing with the most recent studies presented in Table 1. This result is the outcome of a 10-fold cross-validation, which is a very common evaluation approach in the related studies, although we expect a decrease when using a leave-one-out cross-validation, which is a more realistic scenario. It is our intention to advance into such validation scenarios in the near future. For the above results a sampling rate of 20 Hz, a window size of 5 s and an overlap of 80% have been used. These values are proposed as the optimal for this experimental setup. The usage of two independent datasets ensures robustness of the results, always within the limits of each dataset.

For the second optimized feature set the challenge was to correctly classify a set of 16 activities, including falls, with the limitation of the very short duration (<2 s) of some of them, like "stand to sit" and "sit to stand". This resulted into the necessity of reducing the window size for feature extraction with respect to the one used in OFS1. The number of features was reduced as well, striving for a simpler, computationally less demanding, pipeline. The evaluation of this feature set was performed on a subset of MobiAct, not including the activities of the continuous sequences, as well as on the complete dataset. The outcome is encouraging, showing remarkable results on activity recognition and good results in fall recognition. A slight misclassification between the falls was observed. Since it is mainly between the falls, accurate fall detection would be possible with a logical "OR" expression on the classification outcome of the four fall classes. Similar to the evaluation with OFS1, IBk performed better than the J48 decision tree, while the inclusion of scenario-based recorded activities showed practically no deterioration of the average performance of both classifiers based on the F-Measure.

The experimental results obtained indicate that the MobiAct can be considered as a benchmark dataset since it includes a relatively large number of records and a wide range of activities and falls in an easy to manage data format. The latest addition to the dataset, namely the continuous activity sequences expands the suitability of the dataset towards investigating more complex HAR problems including very short activities and uncluttered transitions between activities. Furthermore, since the placement of the smartphone is freely chosen by the subject in any random orientation we believe that it represents real life conditions as close as possible.

The next step towards developing a real-life application requires that (a) orientation data is used in a more efficient manner and (b) assessment and optimization of power consumption (battery usage) requirements for the feature extraction and classification algorithms, is thoroughly studied.

Acknowledgements. The authors gratefully thank all volunteers for their contribution in the production of the MobiAct dataset.

References

1. Vavoulas, G., Chatzaki, C., Malliotakis, T., Pediaditis, M., Tsiknakis, M.: The MobiAct dataset: recognition of activities of daily living using smartphones. In: Proceedings of the International Conference on Information and Communication Technologies for Ageing Well and e-Health, Rome, Italy (2016)
2. Kwapisz, J.R., Weiss, G.M., Moore, S.A.: Activity recognition using cell phone accelerometers. ACM SIGKDD Explor. Newslett. 2(2), 74–82 (2011)
3. Siirtola, P., Röning, J.: Recognizing human activities user-independently on smartphones based on accelerometer data. Int. J. Interact. Multimedia Artif. Intell. 1(5), 38–45 (2012)
4. Khan, A.M., Lee, Y.K., Lee, S.Y., Kim, T.S.: Human activity recognition via an accelerometer-enabled-smartphone using kernel discriminant analysis. In: 5th International Conference in Future Information Technology (FutureTech) (2010)
5. Lee, Y.S., Cho, S.B.: Activity recognition using hierarchical hidden markov models on a smartphone with 3D accelerometer. In: Hybrid Artificial Intelligent Systems, pp. 460–467 (2011)
6. Huq, G.B., Basilakis, J., Maeder, A.: Evaluation of tri-axial accelerometry data of falls for elderly through smart phone. In: ACSW 2016 Proceedings of the Australasian Computer Science Week Multiconference, Canberra, Australia (2016)
7. Vavoulas, G., Pediaditis, M., Chatzaki, C., Spanakis, E.G., Tsiknakis, M.: The MobiFall dataset: fall detection and classification with a smartphone. Int. J. Monit. Surveill. Technol. Res. (IJMSTR) 2(1), 13 (2014)
8. Chatzaki, C., Pediaditis, M., Vavoulas, G., Tsiknakis, M.: Estimating normal and abnormal activities using smartphones. In: 13th International Conference on Wearable, Micro and Nano Technologies for Personalised Health, Crete, Greece (2016)
9. Bayat, A., Pomplun, M., Tran, D.A.: A study on human activity recognition using accelerometer data from smartphones. In: 11th International Conference on Mobile Systems and Pervasive Computing (MobiSPC 2014), vol. 34, pp. 450–457 (2014)
10. Anjum, A., Ilyas, M.U.: Activity recognition using smartphone sensors. In: Consumer Communications and Networking Conference (CCNC), pp. 914–919, 11–14 January 2013
11. Buber, E., Guvensan, A.M.: Discriminative time-domain features for activity recognition on a mobile phone. In: IEEE 9th International Conference on Intelligent Sensors, Sensor Networks and Information Processing (ISSNIP), pp. 1–6, 21–24 April 2014
12. Fan, L., Wang, Z., Wang, H.: Human activity recognition model based on decision tree. In: Proceedings of the 2013 International Conference on Advanced Cloud and Big Data (CBD 2013), pp. 64–68 (2013)
13. Siirtola, P., Roning, J.: Ready-to-use activity recognition for smartphones. In: IEEE Symposium on Computational Intelligence and Data Mining (CIDM), pp. 59–64, 16–19 April 2013
14. Dernbach, S., Das, B., Krishnan, N.C., Thomas, B.L., Cook, D.J.: Simple and complex activity recognition through smart phones. In: 8th International Conference on Intelligent Environments (IE), pp. 214–221, 26–29 June 2012
15. Saputri, T.R.D., Khan, A.M., Lee, S.W.: User-independent activity recognition via three-stage GA-based feature selection. Int. J. Distrib. Sens. Netw. 10(3), 15 (2014)
16. Hung, W., Shen, F., Wu, Y.L., Hor, M.K., Tang, C.Y.: Activity recognition with sensors on mobile devices. In: Proceedings of the 2014 International Conference on Machine Learning and Cybernetics, Lanzhou (2014)

17. Anguita, D., Ghio, A., Oneto, L., Parra, X., Reyes-Ortiz, J.L.: Human activity recognition on smartphones using a multiclass hardware-friendly support vector machine. In: Bravo, J., Hervás, R., Rodríguez, M. (eds.) IWAAL 2012. LNCS, vol. 7657, pp. 216–223. Springer, Heidelberg (2012). doi:10.1007/978-3-642-35395-6_30

18. Anguita, D., Ghio, A., Oneto, L., Parra, X., Reyes-Ortiz, J.-L.: A public domain dataset for human activity recognition using smartphones. In: ESANN 2013 Proceedings, European Symposium on Artificial Neural Networks, Computational Intelligence, Bruges, Belgium (2013)

19. Wang, A., Chuzhou, G., Yang, J., Zhao, S., Chang, C.-Y.: A comparative study on human activity recognition using inertial sensors in a smartphone. IEEE Sens. J. **16**(11), 4566–4578 (2016)

20. Zheng, L., Cai, Y., Lin, Z., Tang, W., Zheng, H., Shi, H., Liao, B., Wang, J.: A novel activity recognition approach based on mobile phone. In: Multimedia and Ubiquitous Engineering, pp. 59–65 (2014)

21. Albert, M.V., Kording, K., Herrmann, M., Jayaraman, A.: Fall classification by machine learning using mobile phones. PLoS ONE **7**(5), e36556 (2012)

22. Zhao, Z., Chen, Y., Wang, S., Chen, Z.: FallAlarm: smart phone based fall detecting and positioning system. Procedia Comput. Sci. **10**, 617–624 (2012)

23. Kansiz, A.O., Guvensan, M.A., Turkmen, H.I.: Selection of time-domain features for fall detection based on supervised learning. Lecture Notes in Engineering and Computer Science, vol. 2208, no. 1, pp. 796–801 (2013)

24. Figueiredo, I.N., Leal, C., Pinto, L., Bolito, J., Lemos, A.: Exploring smartphone sensors for fall detection. J. Mob. User Experience **5**(2), 1–17 (2016)

25. Vavoulas, G., Pediaditis, M., Spanakis, E., Tsiknakis, M.: The MobiFall dataset: an initial evaluation of fall detection algorithms using smartphones. In: IEEE 13th International Conference on Bioinformatics and Bioengineering (BIBE) (2013)

26. Reyes-Ortiz, J.-L., Smartphone-Based Human Activity Recognition. Springer, Switzerland (2015)

27. Leutheuser, H., Schuldhaus, D., Eskofier, B.M.: Hierarchical, multi-sensor based classification of daily life activities: comparison with state-of-the-art algorithms using a benchmark dataset. PLoS ONE **8**(10) (2013)

28. Shoaib, M., Bosch, S., Incel, O.D., Scholten, H.: A survey of online activity recognition using mobile phones. Sensors **15**, 2059–2085 (2015)

29. Reyes-Ortiz, J.-L., Oneto, L., Samà, A., Parra, X., Anguita, D.: Transition-aware human activity recognition using smartphones. Neurocomputing **171**, 754–767 (2016)

30. Hall, M., Frank, E., Holmes, G., Pfahringer, B., Reutemann, P., Witten, I.H.: The WEKA data mining software: an update. ACM SIGKDD Explor. Newsl. **11**(1), 10–18 (2009)

A Self-learning Application Framework for Behavioral Change Support

Ulrich Reimer$^{(\boxtimes)}$, Edith Maier, and Tom Ulmer

Institute for Information and Process Management,
University of Applied Sciences, St. Gallen, Switzerland
{ulrich.reimer,edith.maier,tom.ulmer}@fhsg.ch

Abstract. The paper analyzes current weaknesses of behavioral change support systems such as the lack of adequately taking into account the heterogeneity of target users. Based on this analysis the paper presents an application framework that comprises various components to accommodate user preferences and to adapt system interventions to individual users: a goal hierarchy which users can tailor to their needs, dividing nudges into different types that correspond to speech acts, rules for context-specific triggering of nudges. User adaptation is realized with approaches from user modeling and collaborative filtering. The result is a self-learning application that changes in line with a user's progress, which is expected to enhance user acceptance and increase and sustain people's motivation for behavioral change. The application framework will be evaluated by comparing a mobile health app using the framework with a simplified version of the app that does not support user tailoring and adaptation.

Keywords: Behavioral change support system · Application framework · Nudging · Mobile health · User adaptation · Self-learning · User modeling · Collaborative filtering

1 Introduction

One of the greatest challenges to health systems all over the world is the growing number of people with (multiple) chronic conditions such as diabetes, asthma, cardiovascular disease and obesity. According to the WHO chronic diseases nowadays account for about 80% of the burden of disease [1]. Most of these are lifestyle-related and the risk factors are well-known, including the lack of physical exercise, smoking, a diet rich in fat and sugar, and the excessive consumption of alcohol. Although people are generally aware of the long-term negative consequences, they often lack the motivation as well as the social and emotional support that is required for changing one's behavior.

Besides, we tend to discount long-term gains such as a higher life expectancy and better quality of life in the long run in favor of short-term rewards like the one offered by some delicious cookies. Whilst the majority of the chronically ill may well agree with their doctors' or caregivers' recommendations and fully

© Springer International Publishing AG 2017
C. Röcker et al. (Eds.): ICT4AWE 2016, CCIS 736, pp. 119–139, 2017.
DOI: 10.1007/978-3-319-62704-5_8

intend to adhere to them, e.g. engage in regular exercise and change their diets, they fail to do so. This often results in a value-action gap, i.e. a mismatch between what people say they should do and what they actually do.

Behavioral economics is an approach that rests on the assumption that choices are often made under circumstances of limited rationality and awareness of their implications. When the principles of behavioral economics are implemented into practice, we talk of 'nudging'. Nudging techniques can guide choices through the way in which they are presented. The so-called 'choice architecture' is "intended to provide decision-knowledge through understanding choice-implications and so guiding actions in effective and ethical directions" [2].

Behavioral economics is an approach that also promises to ameliorate the shortcomings of traditional healthcare management, especially with regard to chronic disease (see e.g. [3,4]). Behavioral economists use knowledge from behavioral science as well as motivational psychology and neuroscience to study how individuals make decisions which are often non-rational, and biased by a series of mental shortcuts, for instance, the so-called "status quo bias" [5]. Apart from the status quo bias, people's behavior is also susceptible to the influence of default rules, framing effects and starting points. Consequently, persuasion strategies can involve changing the way options are presented, e.g. by adapting the rules that drive user interaction.

The philosophy of behavioral economics is also called "libertarian paternalism", namely that people should not be forced to act in certain ways, but rather encouraged to act in ways that are better for them or help them stopping bad habits formed over time. This idea of a "gentle push", or "nudge" favors invitations to change behaviors, rather than the introduction of constraints and sanctions to obtain behavior change [6]. Throughout the paper we use the term "nudge" with the following meaning:

Definition:
A *nudge* is a brief persuasive intervention that encourages a specific behavior.

It has been shown that frequent and immediate feedback is very helpful to nudge people towards healthy behavior [7,8]. Mobile devices including smartphones and wearables such as smartwatches offer great opportunities because they can be used for measuring vital parameters such as heart rate, skin conductance or blood pressure but also the number of steps or sleep patterns. Mobile health solutions, i.e. mobile devices connected to medical applications or sensors, can be subsumed under the term 'e-nudging' or 'technological nudging' which according to [2] can be defined as "designing computer systems that augment human decision-making through machine-knowledge and domain-matching, particularly through mobile-device interfaces". The authors have examined how technology can be designed around the principles of libertarian paternalism and developed a conceptual model which integrates users, crowds, web content, micro-education and the cloud-of-things [2].

Most mobile health solutions as well as pure lifestyle apps actually include some kind of support for users to achieve their goals. However, these nudges tend to be hardwired, i.e. they do not adapt to user preferences and needs and on the whole they are not grounded in behavioral change theory (see e.g. [9,10]).

Our recent research therefore focuses on how to use digital technologies to support behavioral change in a systematic way and to allow adaptation to what works best for an individual user. The current article considerably extends an earlier conference paper [11].

2 Components and Challenges of Behavior Change Support Systems

Nudging for healthy behavior using mobile technology has to be viewed in the larger context of so-called behavior change support systems (BCSS) as introduced and defined by Oinas-Kukkonen [12]:

> *"Behavior change support systems (BCSS) are information systems designed to form, alter, or reinforce attitudes or behaviors or both without using coercion or deception."*

The persuasive systems design (PSD) model, a framework for designing a BCSS introduced in [13], draws from the seminal work by Fogg on persuasive technology [14]. It distinguishes two major design steps: first, analyzing the *persuasion context*, second, defining the *BCSS design features*. The persuasion context is defined by the *intent*, the type of change to be achieved, e.g. if it is a one-time or a permanent change, the *event*, which includes the use context as well as the user's goals, and the *strategy*, which determines what kinds of message are to be delivered via which route to the user. The BCSS design features consist of four categories:

primary task support distinguishes various principles of how to support the user, e.g. by reducing complex behavioral goals to smaller goals that can be achieved by simple tasks, or by personalizing the system to the user's specific behavior and preferences;

dialog support deals with how to set up the dialog with the user;

system credibility addresses the issue how to make the system credible for the user;

social support deals with how to improve motivation and adherence by including social influence, e.g. via the peer group, into the system.

Whilst the model suggested by Oinas-Kukkonen already mentions *personalization* as one of many design principles, the concept plays a more important role in more recent work on persuasive systems. However, so far no terminological consensus has emerged. Terms like 'personalization', 'tailoring' and 'user targeting' are used rather interchangeably throughout the literature. For example, [15] use 'tailoring' as an umbrella term with 'personalization' as a sub-concept, whereas op den Akker and his colleagues [16] prefer the terms 'user targeting' and 'adaptation'. They have further elaborated on the PSD model and created a conceptual framework of tailoring which includes the following inter-related key concepts: feedback, inter-human interaction, adaptation, user targeting, goal setting, content awareness, and self-learning. Whilst tailoring techniques such as adaptation and user targeting aim to adapt communication to a user, context-aware systems aim to adapt to a user in a particular context [16].

According to the Dutch researchers, a *self-learning application* is able to update its internal model of the user by recording and learning from the various interactions the user has with the application and thus to change with the user over time. It therefore corresponds to the automatic user adaptation as employed in our BCCS, which also uses other tailoring techniques as defined by [16] such as context awareness, goal setting and user targeting.

In their survey of physical activity monitoring and tailoring they found that most applications only employ feedback – the most obvious form of tailoring – and a few supplement this with an additional technique such as inter-human interaction. They found only one paper [17], which describes the use of more than two different tailoring concepts including user targeting. However, the paper is primarily conceptual in nature and does not provide any detail on technical implementation or algorithms nor does it refer to any behavior change theories.

Op den Akker and his colleagues provide many useful examples of how the above-mentioned concepts are currently being applied and encourage designers of coaching systems to explore different paths or new combinations of tailoring. They also emphasize the need to increase adoption of tailoring methods that are based on behavioral change theories [16]. Although in their article they address real-time physical activity coaching systems, their framework can also be applied to other systems that aim at changing people's behavior.

Whilst there may be no consensus on terminology, authors do agree that it is nearly impossible to design a "one-size-fits-all" system because target user groups are so heterogeneous. In the health domain, for instance, [18] examine individual differences in persuadability and conclude that the intervention of a persuasive system needs to be tailored to the persuasion profile of the specific user. For example, some users react best to strongly persuasive messages while other users respond adversely to too strong an intervention and would require a more low-key suggestion. Prost et al. [19] build upon these results and describe a system that employs personalization based on factors such as persuadability of the user, social-emotional attitude and behavior history. The results of an empirical study on the relationship between personality and the effectiveness of persuasive technologies is presented in [20].

Laverman and his colleagues [21] present an approach to personalizing communication in a BCSS (which they call "self-management support system"). The authors argue that the system should provide information in a way that is "relevant to the user's situation and match[es] the user's preferences and abilities to understand and be persuaded by [it]". The effect of personalizing short text messages to reduce snacking behavior was investigated by Kaptein and his colleagues and the results reported in [22]. A more general overview of the possible roles personalization can play in persuasive systems can be found in [23].

Behavioral change starts with motivation and intent and requires the setting of clear and measurable goals which direct attention and effort toward goal-relevant activities [24]. According to the Goal-Setting Theory, people are more likely to change behavior, the more specific a goal [24]. Results from a review of laboratory and field studies on the effects of goal setting on performance show that in 90% of the studies, specific and challenging goals led to higher performance than easy goals, "do your best" goals, or no goals. Besides, [25] stress that it is important that goals should not just be assigned to a user but that the individual should decide for him/herself if a goal is important to him or her.

Therefore, BCSS include mechanisms for goal setting as well as measuring goal achievement to give appropriate feedback. Many of the smartphone apps that have come into existence as part of the quantified self movement for track-ing and measuring all kinds of activities, support goal setting and typically offer support for achieving these goals, e.g. by giving feedback on current goal achievement, by drawing on peer group support, or by playful competition. In these cases, while goal setting is supported, a user can set only certain types of goals due to the specific focus of these apps, e.g. measuring physical activity, calorie intake, or stress level.

Consequently, while there are many theoretical models available for guiding the proper design of a BCSS and for designing mobile systems for supporting behavioral change in particular, in the end each application has to be hand-crafted and tailored to a specific domain and application scenario. When design-ing a system, developers make assumptions about what will work for the target user group, but once the app has been completed, perhaps even evaluated with a focus group, one cannot but hope that the app will be effective in supporting the intended behavior changes. If this is not the case, it will be very difficult to identify the reasons. Thus, despite the theoretical guidelines available, the actual task of creating a BCSS is more an art than a systematic development process.

One way to tackle this challenge is to devise a more generic BCSS which can be easily configured by the users themselves to meet their needs or which even automatically adapts itself to a user. In this way, fewer assumptions need to be made about the functions that a user actually wants to have.

To this end, we propose mapping the existing theoretical concepts to an *application framework* for creating mobile persuasive systems that can be con-figured to accommodate a wide variety of user requirements without the need to reimplement parts of the system. Additionally, we propose that the framework supports *self-learning* by including components for automatic user adaption dur-ing system runtime.

In our current research we focus on those aspects of the framework which we deem most important for a mobile BCSS and which will help overcome the current shortcomings of mobile health solutions. Our framework therefore

– remedies the limited goal setting capabilities of existing apps by including a *goal hierarchy* that can be set up and edited by a user according to his or her specific needs (maybe together with a person acting as a coach or therapist for the user);

– distinguishes between the ultimate goals a user wants to achieve and the more concrete *operationalized sub-goals* whose achievement can be measured, e.g. with sensors;

– offers a variety of different kinds of persuasive interventions (*nudge types* and *nudge media types*) a user can choose from according to his or her preferences, or which are automatically favored by the system according to their effectiveness for a specific user;

– provides a *rule-based triggering* mechanism for nudges that takes the *user-specific context* into account;

– includes *automatic adaptation mechanisms* that monitor user behavior, correlate system interventions with user behavior and determine which kinds of system interventions work best for a specific user and then adapt its intervention strategy.

In the following section we will describe our framework in more detail.

3   Application Framework for Behavioral Change Support Systems

We are currently implementing our BCSS application framework by adopting a meta modelling approach [26,27]: All constructs that are needed to create a specific BCSS are defined by a *meta model* (cf. Fig. 1). Examples of such constructs are the goal hierarchy and the nudges of different type. A specific BCSS application is represented by an *application model* that is an instance of the meta model. The BCSS is then configured by a user, which results in a user-specific *runtime system* that is an instance of the application model (cf. Fig. 2).

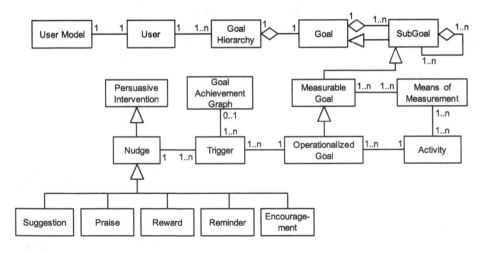

Fig. 1. Core fragment of the BCSS application framework as a meta model.

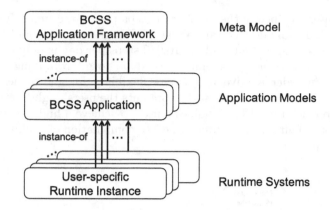

Fig. 2. Model hierarchy.

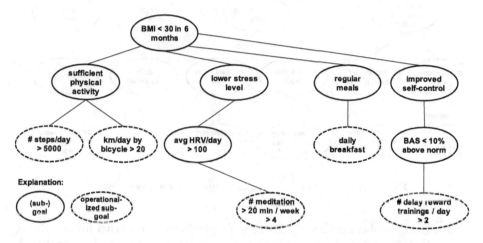

Fig. 3. A user-specific goal hierarchy (runtime level).

For example, the specific BCSS provides various types of goals (Fig. 4) a user can choose from to meet his or her needs and preferences (Fig. 3).

3.1 Goal Hierarchies

At the heart of any BCSS, which also includes mobile health apps, are the goals a user wants to achieve. Goal hierarchies originate in cognitive psychology (e.g. [28]) and play an important role e.g. in interactive systems that create and maintain models of their users' goals and plans. An application framework for creating a BCSS therefore needs to include some mechanism for specifying goals or target behaviors. Many of today's mobile health apps support the setting of user-specific goals but fail to consider the larger context within which these goals are embedded, i.e. what the higher-level goals are. For example, an app might allow users to specify the number of steps per day to make. The higher-level goal behind walking a certain amount of steps per day could be to stay healthy or to lose weight. But walking 10,000 steps per day is only one possible way to achieve this, other possibilities could be to go swimming or cycling. Consequently, in order to give users more flexibility in how to achieve their goals, a *goal hierarchy* is needed which represents the users' higher-level goals as well as how to reach them. This enables a user to achieve a higher-level goal via (a combination of) alternative sub-goals, e.g. a combination of walking, running, cycling and swimming.

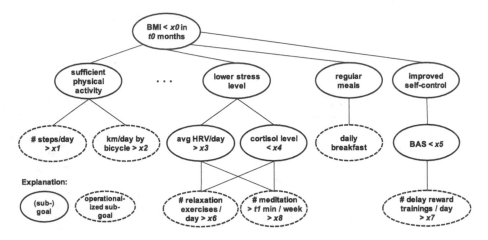

Fig. 4. A goal hierarchy template (application model level).

Our BCSS application framework therefore includes a construct for specifying one or more goal hierarchies for a targeted application domain such as health. A goal hierarchy starts with a top goal which represents a user's primary goal. The top goal tends to be *long-term*, it may be measurable, e.g. "body mass index of below 30 within six months", or be more generic, e.g. "stay healthy". It can usually be achieved by a variety of different ways, e.g. by engaging in physical activity, by lowering the stress level, by eating regular meals or a combination thereof. Each option is represented by a sub-goal. Sub-goals can be broken down into further sub-goals until these can be associated with a measurable activity. We call such goals operationalized:

Definition:
An *operationalized goal* is short-term and is associated with a measurable activity to reach the goal.

Figure 3 shows some examples of operationalized goals. Activities associated with operationalized goals can e.g. be measured via sensors or be entered via diary entries. An activity detection module using a 3D accelerometer and state-of-the-art algorithms can automatically determine if the user is e.g. walking, running, cycling, or climbing stairs, and thus can help to keep track of the achievement of alternative goals for physical activity (see e.g. [29,30]).

Goal hierarchies are set up by a developer of a BCSS to match the intended application domain, such as healthy living or sustainable mobility. At the start, these hierarchies are still templates, specifying what types of goals a user can set. Consequently, the hierarchy templates do not yet contain goals but rather *goal types* which are associated with certain parameters. An example of such a goal type is "physical activity $> x$ steps per day". A user, possibly together with a coach or a therapist, configures the goal hierarchies to his or her needs by selecting goal types and setting values for the goal parameters – goal types are thereby transformed into specific goals. Figure 4 gives an example of a goal hierarchy template with goal types. The goal hierarchy in Fig. 3 has been derived from it.

Users can delete parts of the goal hierarchy so that only the goals they wish to pursue are left. For example, a user who does not like running but prefers cycling would delete the associated sub-goal.

For the time being, we do not permit users to add new types of goals to the predefined goal hierarchy because this would lead to a new application model and might require an additional implementation effort, e.g. to measure the achievement of the added goal. Only if a user were to communicate goal achievement to the BCSS via diary entries could we allow the addition of completely new goal types. This is a possible future extension of our framework.

3.2 Nudge Types

In the course of our research we have conducted extensive interviews with potential end-users which confirm the findings of other researchers [18–20] namely that behavior is influenced by a variety of factors, e.g. age, sex, socio-economic status, attitudes, personality, social environment and peer group. Most existing BCSS, however, have implemented only a fixed or limited set of interventions (or nudges) that do not take into account the *heterogeneity of target users*. This results in low intervention efficacy and low user acceptance.

Nudges have an intent, i.e. they are not just messages but rather actively pursue an aim such as motivating a user to engage in some kind of activity or continue doing so and not give up. This is in line with the theory of *speech acts* as introduced by Austin [31], developed further by Searle [32]. The theory was later picked up by researchers in the area of human-computer interaction to model the interactions between a user and an information system and to align the behavior of the information system with both user history and user context (e.g. [33,34]). The importance of context also applies to a BCSS because the system messages, i.e. the nudges, have to take into account a user's context. We therefore classify nudges into *nudge types* such as suggestions, praises, reminders, rewards, which correspond to speech acts. Together with the construct of goal achievement graphs, we thus create an underlying logic which ensures that generated nudges match the user context (see following section).

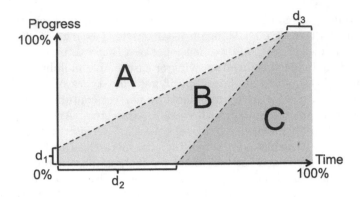

Fig. 5. An initial GA graph for progress-dependent nudges.

Furthermore, nudges can have different *media types*, i.e. they can be textual, visual or audio. A given nudge type can then be realized in different media types. The combination of both offers a wide spectrum of possibilities to accommodate user preferences and to use what works best for a user.

3.3   Goal Achievement Graphs

Having distinguished different nudge types, the next step is to define a mechanism for selecting nudge types according to the user context. We control the triggering of nudges by using *goal achievement graphs* (GA graphs) that relate a user's actual progress to an ideal progress curve. GA graphs make sense for goals which are reached by repeated single activities, such as 10,000 steps per day or self-weighing three times a week. Nudging towards goals with single activities (e.g. self-weighing once per day) is essentially restricted to reminders and thus offers very limited possibilities to support users in achieving their goals. We therefore recommend, whenever possible, to define goals in a way that they are reached by repeated activities.

The rectangular area spanned by a GA graph is divided into the three subareas A, B and C (see Fig. 5): Area A signifies good progress, area B indicates slow progress, while area C indicates that considerable effort is required to achieve the corresponding goal. There is one goal achievement graph for each operationalized sub-goal (cf. the meta model in Fig. 1). The boundaries between the three areas vary depending on when a user typically performs the associated goal achievement activities. Figure 5 shows an initial setup of a GA graph. The two curves which separate the three areas meet at the top with an offset of d_3 to the right margin to make it still possible to reach the goal even when in area C. The offset d_1 lets the user start in area B and thus ensures that he or she will get at least one nudge during the first day, no matter whether the goal has been achieved or missed. Finally, offset d_2 determines when the progress curve falls into area C.

Table 1. Rules for triggering nudges.

Trigger condition	Event type	Nudge type
Area change: from area B to A or from C to B	Catching up	Praise
Area change: from area A to B or from B to C	Lagging behind	Reminder, Suggestion, Encouragement
Percentage of goal reached within area A	Progressing well	Praise
Percentage of goal reached within area B	Lagging behind	Reminder, Suggestion, Encouragement
Percentage of goal reached within area C	Risk of missing goal	Reminder, Suggestion
Percentage of time reached within area A	Progressing well	Praise
Percentage of time reached within area B	Lagging behind	Reminder, Suggestion, Encouragement
Percentage of time reached within area C	Risk of missing goal	Reminder, Suggestion
Time is up within area B	Missed goal narrowly	Encouragement
Time is up within area C	Missed goal by far	Suggestion
Goal reached	Reached goal	Praise, Praise & Suggestion

The goal achievement graphs are used to set triggers for nudges. A variety of *trigger rule schemas* are predefined, e.g. to generate a praise when the user is performing well and progress lies in area A. When progress falls within area B, nudges of different types, such as suggestions or reminders, are triggered. When goal achievement moves into area C, the user is at risk of missing the goal and stronger nudges may be called for than in area B. On the other hand, if the user catches up and moves back into area B or from area B to area A, a praise message may be generated.

Table 1 shows the most important rule schemas for triggering nudges based on goal achievement graphs. The rules consist of a trigger condition which is associated with an event type and a nudge type. A rule does not say exactly which nudge is to be generated but only what kind of nudge. Instead there is a library which contains suitable text messages, visual icons and audio tones for all possible combinations of nudge and event types. Once a rule is triggered and the nudge and event type determined, a suitable nudge is randomly selected and presented in one of a user's preferred media types. Because of the separation between rules on the type level and specific instances of nudges in a library, rule definition is decoupled from individual nudge texts, visuals or tones. As a result, we not only keep the number of rules low but also facilitate the maintenance of a BCSS. This separation is reflected in Tables 1 and 2. The texts in Table 2 make use of variables to refer to the specific goal $G and the associated activity $A. These variables are bound by the triggering rule (not shown).

Table 2. Example texts and visual icons for various event and nudge types.

Event type	Nudge type	Example text/Visual icon
Catching up	Praise	"Congratulations! You're catching up with your goal $G" / Icon: 👍 $G
Lagging behind	Reminder	"Don't forget your goal $G" / Icon: ! $G
Lagging behind	Suggestion	"Let's have a break and do some $A"
Lagging behind	Encouragement	"Your target $G is not yet in reach but you can still make it!"
Progressing well	Praise	"You're making good progress to reach your goal $G!"
Risk of missing goal	Reminder	"You're about to miss your target of $G!
Risk of missing goal	Suggestion	"Why not make some extra effort to still reach your goal $G?"
Missed goal narrowly	Encouragement	"You narrowly missed your goal $G. Next time you'll make it!"
Missed goal by far	Suggestion	"You haven't reached your goal $G. Why not get some support from friends next time?"
Reached goal	Praise	"Congratulations! You've made it: $G" / Icon: 👑 $G
Reached goal	Praise & Suggestion	"Congratulations, you've reached your goal $G! Maybe you can even do more the next time?"

On top of the triggering rules for nudges there is another level of *meta-rules* which control rule triggering. For example, meta rules ensure that there is a minimum time interval between two nudges and to avoid flooding the user with too many nudges.

4   User Adaptation and Self-learning

Personalizing a BCSS to a user's individual needs and preferences requires some effort from the user. As shown by our interviews the average user will shun this additional effort and find it difficult deciding which choices to make, e.g. between alternative ways to reach a goal for physical activity, or which kinds of nudges to prefer. We therefore aim at developing a self-learning system which is able to automatically adapt to the user. Depending on the target of adaptation either user modeling [35] or collaborative filtering [36] is more suitable.

User modeling is based on a user's behavioral history and is independent from other users of the system. It implies the successive build-up of a user model based on user behavior. The user model in turn determines how the system should interact with the user. Adaptation through user modeling is applied to two constructs in our BCSS framework: nudge types and nudge media types (Sect. 4.1) and GA graphs (Sect. 4.2).

Adaptation through *collaborative filtering* draws on the preferences of similar users of the same system and requires a sufficiently large number of users with a sufficiently long history. In our BCSS framework collaborative filtering is employed to recommend goal settings to a user (Sect. 4.3).

4.1 User Modeling: Adapting Nudge Types and Nudge Media Types to Users

Since it has been shown that the intervention of a persuasive system needs to be tailored to a specific user [18] we devised an algorithm to automatically adapt preferred nudge types and nudge media types to users. For example, if a user repeatedly follows a suggestion made by the system, this is a good indicator that the user responds well to suggestion nudges. Also, whilst some users might respond well to reminders or feedbacks that they are falling behind their peer group, other users might simply ignore such messages.

The adaptation is based on which kinds of nudges have proved more successful than others. The system starts by selecting nudge types and nudge media types randomly and monitoring how well each of them works. To this end, the mean progress mp_{nt} a user shows after a nudge of type nt is compared to mp, the user's overall mean progress. If the ratio mp_{nt}/mp is greater than 1, performance after a nudge of type nt is better than overall performance. We call that ratio the impact score of the corresponding nudge type. In the case of nudge media types, we proceed in a similar way.

Nudge types are ranked according to their impact scores. Those with the highest scores are used more often since they (appear to) work better for the particular user. The scores with a value below 1 are used less often. They are not completely blocked because they might work better in the future in which case their scores can increase again.

4.2 User Modeling: Adapting Goal Achievement Graphs

The triggering of nudges by rules that are defined on GA graphs takes the user-specific situation into account and can therefore already be considered a kind of user-specific adaptation. We go beyond that, however, by continuously adapting the boundaries between the three areas in the GA graphs to reflect the user's typical timing of when he or she performs the activities required to reach the corresponding goal. For example, for a user who likes to go running early in the morning, area A would be more to the left and smaller. On the other hand, for a user who usually goes running in the afternoon, area A would stretch more to the right.

We decided to draw the boundary between areas A and B in a way that users stay in the green area A as long as they perform better than their mean progress. The system therefore calculates the boundary between A and B for a given goal g to be the mean of all progress curves from the past where the user achieved the goal g. The first progress curve considered in this calculation is the A-B boundary of the initial graph as shown in Fig. 5.

The definition of the A-B boundary is given by Formulas (1) and (2) and makes use of the function $p_g(i, t)$ which yields the progress (measured in percent) achieved for the operationalized goal g and past interval i from the user history at time t. Past intervals are numbered, e.g. Day 1, Day 2, or Week 1, Week 2. Time t is given in percent of elapsed time within the interval i.

$$AB_g(t) = \frac{1}{n} \sum_{i=1}^{n_g} w_g(i) \cdot ps_g(i, t), \text{ where } n = \sum_{i=1}^{n_g} w_g(i) \tag{1}$$

where $ps_g(i, t)$ yields values only for successful progress curves $p_g(i, t)$ and suppresses unsuccessful ones:

$$ps_g(i, t) = \begin{cases} p_g(i, t): \text{if } p_g(i, 100\%) \geq 100\% \\ 0 \quad : else \end{cases} \tag{2}$$

Since a user's habits may change, the boundaries are calculated using a weighted mean: the weight given to a goal achievement curve gets higher, the more recent the curve, i.e. the higher the interval number i (see Formula (3)). In this way, the GA graphs reflect recent habit changes much faster. To avoid excessive differences between the weights of the oldest and the most recent progress curves, the logarithm used in Formula (3) dampens the increase of the weights for the most recent curves so that their impact does not get too strong.

$$w_g(i) = \frac{1}{log_2(n_g - i + 1) + 1} \tag{3}$$

The B-C boundary is calculated as the mean of all past progress curves that achieved the goal later than the already calculated A-B boundary (see Formula (4)). As with the definition of the A-B boundary, the B-C boundary gives more recent curves a higher weight to better reflect recent habit changes.

$$BC_g(t) = \frac{1}{n} \sum_{i=1}^{n_g} w_g(i) \cdot ps'_g(i, t), \text{ where } n = \sum_{i=1}^{n_g} w_g(i) \tag{4}$$

where $ps'_g(i, t)$ yields values only for successful progress curves $ps_g(i, t)$ that achieved the goal later than the AB_g curve:

$$ps'_g(i, t) = \begin{cases} ps_g(i, t) :\text{if } \exists t', t'' : ps_g(i, t') = 100\% \wedge t' > t'' \wedge AB_g(t'') = 100\% \\ 0 \quad : else \end{cases}$$

An example of an adapted GA graph is given in Fig. 6.

4.3   Collaborative Filtering: Recommendations for Goal Setting

Our BCSS framework makes use of *collaborative filtering* [36] to generate recommendations concerning goal setting, i.e. which operationalized sub-goals to

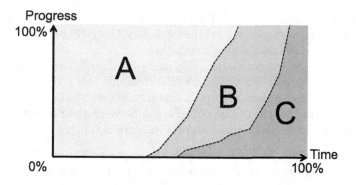

Fig. 6. An adapted GA graph.

pursue to reach a main or higher-level goal and which target values to adopt. Therefore, the recommendations generated for a user u concern:

(a) Sub-goals. For each higher-level goal which a user u shares with another user, the associated operationalized sub-goals with which to achieve it are considered. First a score is calculated for each such sub-goal, then the sub-goals with the highest scores are recommended:

$$score(subgoal) = \frac{1}{1 + n_{sg}} \sum_{i=1}^{n} sim(u, u_i) \cdot has\text{-}subgoal(u_i, subgoal)$$

where

$$has\text{-}subgoal(u, g) = \begin{cases} 1 : \text{if user } u \text{ has subgoal } g \\ 0 : else \end{cases}$$

and

$$n_{sg} = \sum_{i=1}^{n} has\text{-}subgoal(u_i, subgoal)$$

(b) Target Values. For all recommended operationalized sub-goals as well as for operationalized sub-goals already set, a target value is suggested:

$$goal\text{-}value(sgoal, u) = \frac{1}{n_{sg}} \sum_{i=1}^{n} sim(u, u_i) \cdot goal\text{-}value(sgoal, u_i)$$

where $goal\text{-}value(sg, u)$ evaluates to 0 if user u does not have sub-goal sg.

Recommendations are generated only from users with a sufficiently long usage history.

What remains to be discussed is how we define the features with which to describe a user and how to define the similarity measure $sim(u, u')$ on those features. There are two principle approaches for characterizing a user: first, by means of the user's socio-demographic data, and secondly, by his or her past behavior. Clearly, in the case of a BCSS the user's behavior is significantly more relevant than the socio-demographic data. For example, people with different socio-demographic backgrounds are nevertheless likely to behave in a similar way when it comes to maintaining weight loss.

We therefore decided to characterize users by their *behavioral profile*. This includes a profile of basic activities, a workout profile and a stress profile. From all these profiles the system creates a feature vector. Similarity between two users is then defined by the cosine of the angle between their feature vectors. In the following, we look at the three aspects in more detail.

(a) Activity Profile. The BCSS records the user's activities using the sensors connected to the system. For example, with accelerometers it is rather straightforward to detect basic activities such as standing, sitting, walking, running, cycling [29, 30]. The collected activity history is mapped into a *feature vector* which is then used for describing a specific user. For each activity the feature vector includes a value which gives the average percentage of time during a day spent with this particular activity: $\langle t_{avg}(sit), t_{avg}(stand), t_{avg}(walk), t_{avg}(run), t_{avg}(cycle), \ldots \rangle$

(b) Workout Profile. A workout is an activity characterized by physical exertion or a movement or series of movements that tend to be intense. While basic activities can be detected automatically workouts cannot. For example, certain yoga positions might be physically quite exerting but would not generate any significant acceleration which can be measured by an accelerometer. Even if we measured skin temperature or skin conductance, we would not be able to identify a workout since high values for all those parameters can also result from stress. Therefore, the user needs to tell the BCSS the beginning and end of a workout.

The systems determines the intensity of a workout from a user's heart rate (as e.g. measured by a smartwatch), which is recorded whenever the user performs a workout. The heart rate during workouts is measured continuously and for each minute the average value during that minute is calculated. Heart rate values are then aggregated into intervals. We thus obtain a histogram for each day. Since we are not interested in the performance on a particular day but in the average workout performance over a period of time, i.e. the whole user history, we assign the mean value over all days to each bar in the histogram. The histogram consists of six bars which cover the possible ranges of heart rate values. The system adds the y values of each bar in the histogram to the feature vector for describing the workout profile of a user:

$$\langle t_{avg}(bar_1), t_{avg}(bar_2), t_{avg}(bar_3), t_{avg}(bar_4), t_{avg}(bar_5), t_{avg}(bar_6) \rangle$$

Figure 7 shows an example of such a histogram. On the x axis we can see the heart rate intervals, on the y axis we see the associated mean percentages of time per day.

(c) Stress Profile. Finally, we include the user's *stress profile* in the feature vector. The stress profile consists of the average time during a day with high, medium and low stress. For measuring stress levels we build on the results of our SmartCoping project [37] where we have used a chest strap to obtain sufficiently

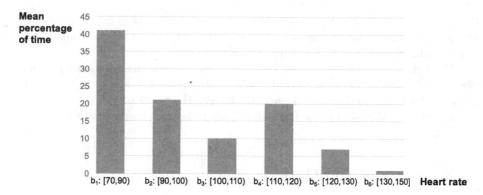

Fig. 7. A histogram for workout features.

reliable measurements of heart rate variability:

$$\langle t_{avg}(high\text{-}stress), t_{avg}(medium\text{-}stress), t_{avg}(low\text{-}stress)\rangle$$

A possible future extension of user adaptation through collaborative filtering would be to include the *success rate of similar users* concerning their main goals. This would imply recommending not only operationalized sub-goals that other users have selected, but those sub-goals that turned out to be most successful in achieving their goals.

5   Evaluation

We are currently implementing the BCSS framework. Subsequently we will conduct an evaluation with people who wish to reduce their weight or maintain their previously achieved weight loss. To this end, we are developing a smartphone app which is based on our framework and offers a variety of weight-related goals, including physical activity, self-weighing, eating behavior and calorie intake.

The app will be distributed via the Apple AppStore, which will help to reach a large number of users. This is important for the study because the collaborative filtering algorithms of our system, in particular, require large numbers of users to be effective. We will utilize the templates offered by the Apple ResearchKit to take care of issues such as seeking informed consent and giving participants control over what data they want to share. According to our study design, users will have to agree that they get one of two app versions without knowing which version they get. Nor do they know in which respects the two versions differ. This is important for randomized control and also to avoid bias.

The *static version* of the app reflects the standards of BCSS currently available, i.e. the version has a set of predefined goals and fixed interventions. The interventions include a reduced set of nudge types which are hardwired and not adaptable to the user. Nudges are triggered at fixed time intervals and for fixed amounts of progress, e.g. a positive and praising nudge whenever 80% of the goal is reached and an encouraging nudge whenever progress is below 50% at 80% of the time. The *dynamic and self-learning version* contains all the components and adaptation algorithms described in this paper.

The primary *outcome measure* of the study is goal achievement: (a) percentage of achieved operationalized goals, and (b) the average time needed to achieve the goals. According to our hypothesis, the users of the dynamic and self-learning version should perform significantly better than users of the static version.

6   Conclusions and Outlook

In this paper we have presented an application framework for behavioral change support systems (BCSS) that comprises various components for tailoring a BCSS to users' needs and preferences. One of these components is a *goal hierarchy* which can be set up to represent the goals a user wants to achieve. The higher-level goals (e.g. reaching a BMI below 30 in six months) can be broken down into more specific goals that are operationalized, i.e. can be achieved by associated measurable activities.

The application framework further distinguishes different types of persuasive interventions, which we call nudges. These *nudge types* correspond to speech acts and play a crucial role in ensuring that a generated nudge matches the user context. We have introduced the construct of *goal achievement graphs* for selecting nudge types according to the user context, e.g. if a user is lagging behind or catching up.

To do justice to the heterogeneity of target users, our framework includes self-learning components for *automatically adapting system interactions* to users' needs and preferences as well as their changing behavior. For this purpose, we have presented *user modeling* approaches that take into account a user's behavioral history as well as *collaborative filtering* techniques that draw on the collected evidence from other users of the system. Together, these result in user-specific nudges as well as recommendations concerning setting one's goals and how best to achieve them.

The constructs of the application framework as well as the adaptation algorithms will be *evaluated* by comparing a mobile health app implemented with the framework with a simplified version of the app that does not support individual goal setting, only has fixed nudges and lacks user adaptation.

In the future, we will integrate constructs for social support and further nudge types, e.g. for playful competition, into our framework. We are also planning to embed the framework into a more general approach where the activities associated with operationalized sub-goals are chosen from the predictors of a predictive model. For example, long-term studies have shown that regular self-weighing and having breakfast regularly are strong predictors for weight loss and weight-loss maintenance (see e.g. [38]). Such predictors would therefore be included as *evidence-based goals* in the goal hierarchy. In this scenario, a therapist familiar with such predictors co-decides with a user which goals to set.

Finally, we are considering applying our BCSS framework to domains other than health, e.g. to mobility. Here, the main goal consists in achieving a smaller ecological footprint which is to be reached by encouraging users to use public transport or cycle to work [39].

Acknowledgements. The research presented in this paper has been made possible by a grant from Gebert Rüf Foundation. Our thanks go also to the members of a student group for their contributions to this research: M. Eggenschwiler, S. Frigg and R. Zuberbühler.

References

1. World Health Organization: Global Health Estimates: Deaths, disability-adjusted life year (DALYs), years of life lost (YLL) and years lost due to disability (YLD) by cause, age and sex, 2000–2012 (2012)
2. Thomas, A.M., Parkinson, J., Moore, P., Goodman, A., Xhafa, F., Barolli, L.: Nudging through technology: choice architectures and the mobile information revolution. In: Proceedings Eighth International Conference on P2P, Parallel, Grid, Cloud and Internet Computing, pp. 255–261 (2013)
3. Cabinet Office: Applying behavioural insight to health. Institute for Government, UK (2010)
4. European Commission: Green paper on mobile health (2014)
5. Kahneman, D.: Thinking, Fast and Slow. Penguin Books, New York (2011)
6. Thaler, R.H., Sunstein, C.R.: Nudge: Improving Decisions About Health, Wealth, and Happiness. Penguin Books, New York (2009)
7. Loewenstein, G., Asch, D.A., Volpp, K.G.: Behavioral economics holds potential to deliver better results for patients, insurers, and employers. Health Aff. **32**, 1244–1250 (2013)
8. Maier, E., Ziegler, E.: Sanfte Stupser für gesundheitsförderliches Verhalten - oder Nudging im Gesundheitswesen. Clinicum **3–15**, 76–81 (2015)
9. Lister, C., West, J.H., Cannon, B., Sax, T., Brodegard, D., Eysenbach, G.: Just a fad? Gamification in health and fitness apps. JMIR Serious Games **2**, e9 (2014)
10. Patel, M., Asch, D., Volpp, K.: Wearable devices as facilitators, not drivers, of health behavior change. J. Am. Med. Assoc. **313**, 459–460 (2015)
11. Reimer, U., Maier, E.: An application framework for personalised and adaptive behavioural change support systems. In: Proceedings of 2nd International Conference on Information and Communication Technologies for Ageing Well and e-Health (ICT4AWE) (2016)
12. Oinas-Kukkonen, H.: Behavior change support systems: the next frontier for Web science. In: Proceedings of the Web Science Conference 2010 (2010)
13. Oinas-Kukkonen, H., Harjumaa, M.: Persuasive systems design: key issues, process model, and system features. Commun. Assoc. Inform. Syst. **24**, 28 (2009)
14. Fogg, B.J.: Persuasive Technology: Using Computers to Change What We Think and Do. Morgan Kaufmann, San Francisco (2002)
15. Hawkins, R.P., Kreuter, M., Resnicow, K., Fishbein, M., Dijkstra, A.: Understanding tailoring in communicating about health. Health Educ. Res. **23**, 454–466 (2008)
16. op den Akker, H., Jones, V.M., Hermens, H.J.: Tailoring real-time physical activity coaching systems: a literature survey and model. User Model. User-Adap. Inter. **24**, 351–392 (2014)

17. Bielik, P., Tomlein, M., Krátky, P., Mitrík, Š., Barla, M., Bieliková, M.: Move2Play: an innovative approach to encouraging people to be more physically active. In: Proceedings of the 2nd ACM SIGHIT International Health Informatics Symposium, pp. 61–70. ACM (2012)

18. Kaptein, M., Lacroix, J., Saini, P.: Individual differences in persuadability in the health promotion domain. In: Ploug, T., Hasle, P., Oinas-Kukkonen, H. (eds.) PERSUASIVE 2010. LNCS, vol. 6137, pp. 94–105. Springer, Heidelberg (2010). doi:10.1007/978-3-642-13226-1_11

19. Prost, S., Schrammel, J., Röderer, K., Tscheligi, M.: Contextualise! Personalise! Persuade! A mobile HCI framework for behaviour change support systems. In: Proceedings of the 15th International Conference on Human-computer Interaction with Mobile Devices and Services, pp. 510–515. ACM, New York (2013)

20. Halko, S., Kientz, J.A.: Personality and persuasive technology: an exploratory study on health-promoting mobile applications. In: Ploug, T., Hasle, P., Oinas-Kukkonen, H. (eds.) PERSUASIVE 2010. LNCS, vol. 6137, pp. 150–161. Springer, Heidelberg (2010). doi:10.1007/978-3-642-13226-1_16

21. Laverman, M., Neerincx, M.A., Alpay, L.L., Rövekamp, T.A., Schonk, B.J.: How to Develop Personalized eHealth for Behavioural Change: Method & Example. Technical report TNO 2014, R10758 (2014)

22. Kaptein, M., De Ruyter, B., Markopoulos, P., Aarts, E.: Adaptive persuasive systems: A study of tailored persuasive text messages to reduce snacking. ACM Trans. Interact. Intell. Syst. 2, 10: 1–10: 25 (2012)

23. Berkovsky, S., Freyne, J., Oinas-Kukkonen, H.: Influencing individually: fusing personalization and persuasion. ACM Trans. Interact. Intell. Syst. 2, 9:1–9:8 (2012)

24. Locke, E., Latham, G.: Building a practically useful theory of goal setting and task motivation: a 35-year odyssey. Am. Psychol. 57, 705 (2002)

25. Consolvo, S., Klasnja, P., McDonald, D.W., Landay, J.A.: Goal-setting considerations for persuasive technologies that encourage physical activity. In: Proceedings of the 4th International Conference on Persuasive Technology, ACM, pp. 8:1–8:8 (2009)

26. Karagiannis, D., Kühn, H.: Metamodelling platforms. In: Bauknecht, K., Tjoa, A.M., Quirchmayr, G. (eds.) EC-Web 2002. LNCS, vol. 2455, pp. 182–182. Springer, Heidelberg (2002). doi:10.1007/3-540-45705-4_19

27. Atkinson, C., Kühne, T.: Model-driven development: a metamodeling foundation. IEEE Softw. 20, 36–41 (2003)

28. Schank, R.C., Abelson, R.P.: Scripts, Plans, Goals and Understanding: An Inquiry into Human Knowledge Structures. Lawrence Erlbaum, Hillsdale (1977)

29. Kwapisz, J.R., Weiss, G.M., Moore, S.A.: Activity recognition using cell phone accelerometers. SIGKDD Explorations Newsl. 12, 74–82 (2011)

30. Slim, S.O., Atia, A., Mostafa, M.-S.M.: An experimental comparison between seven classification algorithms for activity recognition. In: Gaber, T., Hassanien, A.E., El-Bendary, N., Dey, N. (eds.) The 1st International Conference on Advanced Intelligent System and Informatics (AISI2015), November 28-30, 2015, Beni Suef, Egypt. AISC, vol. 407, pp. 37–46. Springer, Cham (2016). doi:10.1007/978-3-319-26690-9_4

31. Austin, J.L.: How to Do Things with Words. Oxford University Press, Oxford (1962)

32. Searle, J.: Speech Acts. Cambridge University Press, Cambridge (1969)

33. Winograd, T., Flores, F.: Understanding Computers and Cognition. Ablex Publishing Corp, Norwood (1986)

34. Lehtinen, E., Lyytinen, K.: Action based model of information system. Inform. Syst. **11**, 299–317 (1986)
35. Kobsa, A.: Generic user modeling systems. User Model. User-Adap. Inter. **11**, 49–63 (2001)
36. Adomavicius, G., Tuzhilin, A.: Toward the next generation of recommender systems: a survey of the state-of-the-art and possible extensions. IEEE Trans. Knowl. Data Eng. **17**, 734–749 (2005)
37. Reimer, U., Maier, E., Laurenzi, E., Ulmer, T.: Mobile stress recognition and relaxation support with SmartCoping: user adaptive interpretation of physiological stress parameters. In: Proceedings Hawaii International Conference on System Sciences (HICSS-50) (2017)
38. Feller, S., Müller, A., Mayr, A., Engeli, S., Hilbert, A., de Zwaan, M.: What distinguishes weight loss maintainers of the german weight control registry from the general population? Obesity **23**, 1112–1118 (2015)
39. Maier, E.: Smart mobility - encouraging sustainable mobility behaviour by designing and implementing policies. JeDEM-eJournal of eDemocracy and Open Government **4**, 115–141 (2012)

Author Index

Printed in the United States
By Bookmasters